The Science of Weight Loss

The honest truth about how to lose weight

John Josefson

Contents

CHAPTER 1

Introduction

If you're looking for an easy way to lose weight, then this book isn't for you. There are, quite literally, a thousand and one such books out there. But most of those books doesn't make sense. They tell you that you can lose weight by eating only a certain vegetable, getting rid of certain food products, lowering the amount of butter on each sandwitch, substituting one food for another, drinking light beverages, and so on.

Most of that won't help you if you're trying to lose weight in the long term. If you really want to lose weight, then this is the only thing you really need to know:

▶ If you eat more calories than you use, you gain weight.

▶ If you eat less calories than you use, you lose weight.

All of the diets mentioned have this in common. They might not tell you outright, but that's what it all comes down to. One famous diet is the orange diet, where you substitute one meal a day wth an orange. Not so much because the orange in particular is a useful substitute, but because it lowers the calorie intake by almost one meal a day.

Keeping this in mind as you read this book will help you understand how you can lose weight, and keep your weight constant. This book will take you through the science of weightloss. We'll talk about what is happening in your body as you lose weight, how you burn calories and how the food you eat turns into calories.

If you follow some very simple guidlines, you'll soon start losing weight, and always keep in mind, that the calories you take into your body, needs to be less or equal to the calories your body uses. If it's not, you gain weight. If they are, you lose weight.

Let's start losing weight!

CHAPTER 2

What Happens in Your Body when You Lose Weight?

What happens inside of your body when you lose weight? It may be a topic that you have never considered before. Certainly you have considered what happens on the outside of your body as you lose weight. It is a much harder thing to ignore. Some parts of your body seem to shrink and morph into different forms. You may rediscover some muscles or bone protrusions that you haven't seen in a long while. Shirts hang differently from your shoulders. Pants allow for additional movement and breathing room. Walking up the stairs is less tiring. Touching your toes is definitely more feasible. Your skin generally adjusts to your new body.

Many people claim additional benefits after they lose weight.

They say that they feel more energetic. Some people claim to fall asleep more quickly and then sleep more deeply. They may even say that they are more able to concentrate on their work, or that their asthma doesn't act up as much as it used to.

Are these truly possible effects of weight loss? If so, then there must be some other things going on inside your body as you lose weight. The outside effects are what you notice first, but what goes on inside of your body is much more complex and interesting.

Below the skin over your entire body, there is a layer of fat cells. In science-lingo they are referred to as "adipocytes," which does sound a little more appetizing than "fat cells." In some areas of your body, such as your forehead or feet, the layer of adipocytes is very thin, but it is still there. It is biologically necessary to have this layer of fat cells everywhere from your eyelids to your fingers to the tops of your feet. Without the layer of adipose tissue, your body would not be able to regulate its temperature. You could die from hypothermia. These insulating cells help to avoid wasting excessive calories heating and reheating your body. The layer of adipocytes also protects your organs from injury. When elbows are thrown in a pick-up basketball game, it is unlikely that any internal organs will be punctured. (Again, this is all just part of your body's very smart plan to survive.)

So there is a certain amount of adipose tissue that is necessary to keep you healthy, warm, and injury-free. There is a third use for the fat cells, one that isn't a biological necessity like your stay-warm fat and your protective fat are. This third type of fat is stored fat. The body will attempt to accumulate as many extra calories as possible in the adipocytes, just in case famine conditions suddenly arose in the United States. Adipose tissue is the body's storage area for extra energy that you might be able to use some day. This stockpiling trait might not be so nice to have when you are in a land of plenty, but it has helped humans survive for lots of years through rougher times.

The extra fat that goes in storage will be placed in a predictable pattern. If you are like everyone else on the planet, fat probably won't be stashed over your shins or under your scalp. There are adipocytes there, but it's just not practical. In some other areas of the body, there is a much more generous layer of adipocytes, and physically there is a lot more possibility for expansion. Your stomach, waist, backside, and legs are prime examples. You may be able to come up with an even more comprehensive list from personal experience.

These specific storage areas of the body have the ability to store many adipocytes, and these adipocytes have the ability to expand almost indefinitely. As extra body fat is accumulated, they can accommodate more and more. The cells themselves have a stretchable structure, expanding and shrinking as the body adds or takes away fat. It's kind of an ingenious design, if you think about it.

As a person loses their extra weight, the larger, expanded

adipocytes will be forced to give up some of their fat stores and return to their original size. They will remain in the adipose tissue as functioning cells, ready to expand again at a moment's notice so that the body will never be forced to waste precious energy that it may come by.

In the initial stages of weight loss, about three-quarters of the weight lost comes out of the fat tissues. The rest comes from other lean tissues in the body, like muscles, and possibly bone tissue. Muscle cells are made from proteins filled up with water; that's why muscle tissue weighs so much. Muscle cells also require more energy to maintain than fat cells. When weight loss begins because the body is given fewer calories than it is used to, the body is "scared" into giving up some of the muscle tissue. It is just trying to conserve in case the calorie deprivation is long-term.

Many people refer to the loss of muscle as "losing water weight." To lose more fat and less water weight, it is important to lose weight gradually. After you have been involved in the weight loss process for a couple of weeks, the proportion shifts more in your favor. Closer to 90% of the weight lost will be fat, and only 10% or so will come from lean tissues. This is a strong argument for making long-term, minor diet and lifestyle changes instead of going for the two-week quick-fix juice diet.

The actual shrinking of the adipocytes is what causes many of the aforementioned outwardly visible effects of weight loss. That makes sense enough; if you had had to guess what was going on in there, you probably would have suspected something similar.

But unfortunately, the adipocytes are not just a benign bunch of extra baggage. Because of their influence on the body, reduction of fat tissue is merely the beginning of a chain of physical events that starts when weight loss occurs. Some of the effects of weight loss are not initially apparent, but are quite possibly the most valuable. These changes are made possible because of the biological role of fat in the body.

Adipocytes are responsible for other activities besides just storing calories for a rainy day. One of their most important side jobs is giving off certain hormones related to hunger, the feeling of fullness, and digestion. The larger the amount of adipose tissue that is present in the body, the more of these hormones that are released into your bloodstream to communicate with other organs. The opposite is also true.

As you can imagine, this can affect the functioning of quite a few systems in the body. All of the effects caused by the extra fat tissue are not completely understood by modern science. There are quite a few researchers are working on this question right now to better understand why exactly it is that being overweight increases the risk for so many ailments. They would like to figure out in detail what role the hormones have to play in the whole process.

Another way that the amount of adipocytes in your body can

contribute to other problems is that it changes the physics of your body mechanics. The physics of gravity and the pull of different forces applies just as much to the human body as it does to buildings and bridges. Your body puts the extra weight in the least-intrusive position possible: close to the center, spread out as much as possible, but it is still an extra strain on the frame of your body. The weight of the fat pockets pulls in unnatural ways on your joints and spine. If you have gained weight, then you will probably have to move differently, walk differently, and sit differently. The alignment of bones is pushed around and stress on tendons and ligaments in increased in bad ways.

Finally, when a person is overweight, their body size grows, but their internal organs do not. This puts their heart, lungs, liver, and everything else into overdrive trying to maintain and supply the needs of more body mass than they were intended to care for. Some of the diseases associated with gaining weight may be due to "wear and tear" type problems. Your organs do need regular exercise, but this chronic tyrannical overworking can cause them to revolt.

Predictably, all of these effects (hormonal, mechanical, and physical) of extra adipose tissue have far-reaching consequences for long-term health. The risk for developing Type II (also known as adult-onset) Diabetes increases when you are overweight or obese. With an effect that drastic on your health, you might assume that a person has to gain a lot of weight to increase their risk for diabetes, but it's simply not true. Gaining between eleven and eighteen pounds makes your risk for diabetes double the risk for other people like you who have not gained any weight. The biological effect of an extra ten pounds is amazingly significant, and unfortunately you can't hide it away in a more flattering outfit. The risk still increases, because of the biological activity of the fat cells.

For someone who is already diabetic, extra weight will probably make it harder for him or her to control daily blood sugar levels. That's pretty alarming, because good blood sugar control is very important. It's the only way to prevent diabetes complications like blindness and circulation problems that can result in amputations.

Weight gain also has several effects related to the heart and heart disease. High blood pressure is twice as common in overweight people as in people considered to be a healthy weight. High blood pressure contributes to the risk for heart disease. It occurs when there is a lot of resistance in the body to normal blood circulation. If someone has high blood pressure, it means that it is more difficult for his or her heart to pump. So there is extra strain on each and every beat.

Cholesterol and triglycerides in the blood are also intrinsically related to heart disease, and they are another area where the numbers tend to increase as weight is gained. Furthermore, the amount of "bad cholesterol" tends to be higher in overweight individuals, and the amount of "good cholesterol" tends to be lower. Gaining weight seems to be an overall bad deal when it comes to blood lipid levels, which in turn directly affect the heart. You are also at a higher risk for Chronic Venous Insufficiency, which, as you may have surmised from the name of the condition, is not a good thing. Strokes, which are also related to blood circulation and clots, are also more likely if you gain weight.

You are also more likely to develop several types of cancers. Included in this list are endometrial cancer, breast cancer, colon cancer, gallbladder cancer, prostate cancer, kidney cancer, and esophageal cancer. Several diseases are more prevalent in the overweight and obese populations. This includes things like gout, incontinence, gallbladder disease, cirrhosis, and acute hepatitis.

The mechanical changes in your posture and movements over time are the cause of many more physical problems. If you are overweight, you are much more likely to have osteoarthritis and/or rheumatoid arthritis. In fact, for every two pounds that you gain, you are nine to thirteen percent more likely to develop arthritis.

There is a higher risk for carpal tunnel and for lower back pain. There is a good chance that you will suffer from general joint or muscle pains as well. The chronic stress on your knees makes you more susceptible to damaging these joints and requiring knee replacement surgery. That is, of course, expensive, painful, and requires a long recovery and rehabilitation period, but the worst part is that being overweight makes you more likely to have complications during surgery. Your immune system typically doesn't function as effectively as someone of a healthy weight, and so there is a higher risk for infections while your wounds heal. And the final kicker is that your joint replacements are actually more likely to wear out and need replaced again because you are subjecting them to the same forces that caused your natural knees to go.

You may find that extra weight affects your breathing. Many respiratory problems are linked to obesity, like sleep apnea and asthma. Many people find notable relief from these diseases after they lose some weight.

Overweight women can have a host of reproductive problems, from conception through delivery. Just as regular diabetes is a risk general health risk, overweight women run the risk of getting gestational diabetes during pregnancy. Many overweight women find that they are less fertile than when they are a healthier weight. If they do become pregnant while overweight, both their own as well as their child's risk for death increase. This clearly doesn't affect everyone; it is just that the total risk increases. Overweight women are ten times more likely to develop high blood pressure during pregnancy than women of a healthy weight. Their babies are more likely to be born bigger, meaning that more C-sections are required, and are more likely to have low blood sugar, which can cause brain damage and seizures. The babies also have a higher chance of birth defects, especially neural tube defects. Taking folic acid helps to reduce this type of birth defects, but some studies show that the reduction is not as strong in overweight women.

So that may seem like a long list of bad news for someone who is looking to lose weight. But there is corresponding good news! Many of these health risks are entirely reversible. How can you do that? Send your body through the opposite process; lose the weight that you have gained. As you lose weight, the fat will be taken out of the adipocytes. They will shrink down, and as their presence becomes a smaller and smaller percentage of your total body weight, they will do less damage. Less hormones will be released to mess with everything else. There will be less strain on your vital organs; less work for them each day means less burnout overall. Your posture and movement will be corrected. Taking away the extra pull will alleviate some aches and pains. Your knees will love you.

On the disease front, your risk for diabetes goes way down. If you were already diabetic before your weight loss, you may find it easier to control your diabetes, and may require less medication. The risk diminishes for endometrial cancer, breast cancer, colon cancer, gallbladder cancer, prostate cancer, kidney cancer, esophageal cancer, gout, incontinence, gallbladder disease, cirrhosis, and acute hepatitis.

Your lipid panel will get better; cholesterol and triglycerides will go down. This will save you not only in terms of reducing your risk of heart attack, but also time-wise when you go to the doctor for your annual physical. Think of the amount of time that is usually spent on the "health lecture." (That would be when the doctor sighs and starts suggesting that you really need to lose some weight, etc, etc.) Wouldn't it be great to go in, get examined, and have your doctor instead tell you that you look great and should keep up whatever you are doing?

Achieving these health benefits is not some remote possibility. Losing only five to fifteen percent of your body weight can go a long way to reduce your overall health risks, especially heart disease. You can definitely do that; think of the return on your investment! It's a steal.

The crazy thing is that the above list didn't even factor in the beneficial changes that come from eating fruits and vegetables and exercising, which, let's face it, is how you're going to be able to lose the weight anyway. If you lose weight through these methods, your risk for cancer and heart disease goes down even more. It's like a buy-one, get-one-free sale on longevity.

So try not to be overwhelmed. Now that you have a much more detailed idea of the cascading changes in your body that begin with weight loss, make the decision to get some of those changes started in your own body!

CHAPTER 3

How Food is turned into Calories

You probably know that all foods contain calories, and that's how you get energy. But do you know how the calories were put there in the first place? The energy that you get from a calorie originally came from the sun. Through photosynthesis plants capture the heat and light energy that comes down from the sun and make chemical bonds to hold the energy. When we eat a plant, we ingest the chemical bonds that contain this energy source.

Our bodies have methods to transfer the energy to our own cells or store the energy for later use. If an animal eats the plant, it also incorporates the energy from the plant into its body as we humans do. We could choose to eat an animal instead of a plant. It is a little bit different than eating the plant, but we still get those same energy-containing chemical bonds, which is the purpose of eating in the first place!

The human body uses this valuable energy to power many different processes necessary to life. They can be generally classified into four categories: making chemical compounds, moving our bodies, sending electrical impulses, and balancing ion concentration. These are the human uses for calories on the most basic level.

The first body process to require calories is the manufacture of chemical compounds in the body. Our bodies frequently take one chemical and make it into another one to better suit its purposes. Some chemicals are stored in one form, and then they are converted to a different form once they are needed. It might sound inefficient, but in some cases it can be necessary.

A good example is digestive juice. The stomach has a special lining with a lot of mucus to be able to withstand the power of this very acidic fluid. However, the juice itself is produced in some nearby glands that do not have this protective power. They could hardly hold the digestive juice for hours, just waiting for you to eat something. Instead, the juice is made into a non-acidic form in the glands. It waits there until needed in the digestion process, when the body chemically converts it as needed. This is just one of many possible examples of situations in which the body uses energy to make chemical compounds.

The second use of energy by the body is for body movement. Typing with your hands, rolling your eyes, and tapping your toes all require calories. This is probably the most self-explanatory use of calories; most people are aware that calories provide the energy power needed for actions. To be able to contract your leg muscles in sync as you walk, your body will need to use some energy.

A related, but distinct, use of energy is that used for electrical nervous transmissions. To communicate with your whole body and to control all of your appendages, your brain sends electrical impulses out through your nervous system. Electrical messages are constantly being sent and they are needed for almost everything. The nervous system controls all of the action in the body, from digestion to hand-to-eye coordination, and the preferred method of intra-body communication is through electrical impulses. This messaging system isn't free. We need a certain amount of calories to make it happen every day.

The last category of your body's calorie expenditure is used to balance the ion concentrations throughout your body. A lot of the cells are very sensitive to changes in percentage of sodium, potassium, etc. Changing the concentration of various ions within the cell can be fatal. In order to prevent problems, the human body has an intricate system of boundaries at the edges of the cells. In many cases, little pumps are at work pushing ions to one side or the other. There is constant, round-the-clock pumping at the boundary of your cell walls to maintain the ideal levels. This optimizes the hydration and functioning of different cells in the body, but still costs calories.

In order to continue functioning smoothly in regards to manufacturing chemical compounds, performing body movements, sending electrical nerve transmissions, and balancing ion concentration, your body has a highly specialized method of extracting the calories from the food. In lay terms, we call it "digestion."

So here's how the food is actually processed and used by your body. Say you go through the late-night drive-thru for a couple of burritos and a coke. Or maybe you are on lunch break at work and you grab something from the vending machine. Or this example could even involve the last home-cooked meal that your mom made for you. All of these meals are basically comprised of four basic chemical elements: carbohydrates, fat, protein, and/or alcohol.

There are no other chemical substances that can give us calories. Scientists have developed some sugar alcohols, which are low-calorie sweeteners that are used in things like chewing gum, but your basic four (carbohydrates, fats, proteins, and alcohols) are what it all started with. Each of these nutrients has a slightly different function in the body; all of them are necessary. It's always suspicious when a diet tries to exclude any particular one of the main nutrients, because they so clearly work well together.

Carbohydrates, protein, fat, and alcohol are chemically different. They will each take a slightly different route through digestion, but each one eventually results in net calories ready to be used. These are the only substances that can provide you with calories. Everything else is a waste of your chewing effort.

So you sit down with your food (or drive down the road, whichever the case may be.) You go through the traditional chew, chew, chew, and swallow technique, which doesn't at all require a detailed description. At this point, the chewed-up food makes its way down your esophagus into your stomach. The conditions in your stomach are pretty rough. The pH typically stays less than 2, thanks to the stomach acid mentioned earlier.

The acidity of the stomach is what breaks the food up into smaller parts. Proteins are broken up into amino acids. Carbohydrates are broken up into single sugar molecules. Fats are broken up into smaller fats. Alcohols are not changed in the stomach. Because they are fat-soluble, they pass directly through the lining of your stomach and into your bloodstream in a matter of minutes.

If you have eaten a lot of other food along with the alcohol, the alcohol spends some time mixed up with the carbohydrates, fats, and proteins, and so it is slower to go into your bloodstream. If you drink alcohol on an empty stomach, it is metabolized much more quickly. You may have had personal experiences with this phenomenon.

The three nutrients that remain in your stomach after the

alcohol has been absorbed into the bloodstream continue to mix with the stomach acid for a couple more hours until they are completely broken into their basic elements and are all together in a thick liquid called chyme. The chyme moves on to your small intestine for digestion.

Some people feel deceived when they realize that your small intestine does the real digestion work, not your stomach. It's not as flashy, but it gets the job done. The cells of the small intestine don't have smooth walls, but rather, walls with lots of tentacle-like things called villi. The villi greatly increase the total surface area of the small intestine to maximize the absorption of nutrients.

The amino acids and sugars that are absorbed through the walls of the small intestine go directly into the bloodstream. The fats are also absorbed through the small intestine, but take a less direct route to the bloodstream. The fats are first conducted through the lymphatic system and then go into the blood as well. The intestines also absorb various vitamins and minerals. They are necessary, but don't provide any calories.

Some people have lost parts of their intestines at some point in their lives. This could have been caused by many different things, including radiation treatments for cancers in the intestines or radiation of other nearby organs, the removal of part of the intestine, for whatever reason, or other problems. Parts of the intestines can also be lost during some types of bariatric surgery. If any patient has any missing intestine, or if their intestines have lost the ability to absorb vitamins and minerals, then heavy supplements or even injected vitamins will be prescribed. Normally, this will be something that is required for the rest of the patient's life.

Once digestion is over, the body has already captured the majority of protein, carbohydrates, fat, vitamins, and minerals that were present in the food. At this point after digestion, your blood steam is thick with sugars, proteins, and fats ready to be used by the body. When someone is fed by IV in a hospital, they are essentially just jumping directly to this step of the process. The bags of feeding solution are carefully balanced to contain broken-down fats, carbohydrates, and proteins in the ideal proportions.

You can also think about the digested food in your bloodstream with regards to blood tests. Your doctor makes you fast before getting blood drawn for a cholesterol test because the cholesterol standards are based on the amounts of fats that circulate through your body all the time. If you have eaten before your test, then the fat will still be in your blood and you will get a "high" cholesterol reading.

Something has to prompt the circulating nutrients to leave the bloodstream. They don't really do anything there anyway (except mess up your cholesterol tests.) What happens is that hormones are released that will carry the various nutrients to cells where they can be used.

One of the most famous of these hormones is insulin, the

one that carries the sugars. In diabetics, there is a either a problem with the production of insulin or a problem with the ability of the insulin to carry the sugars into the cells. Without enough functioning insulin, the sugars stay in the bloodstream, making it thick and slow. This is the cause of complications with circulation in diabetics.

After the hormones carry the proteins, fat, and carbohydrates to the cells, the body begins to use these materials for projects all over. First, proteins are taken to rebuild tissues in the body. Only proteins can be used for this. Any leftover proteins will be chemically changed into sugars and used as energy. This is why most people don't need protein shakes. Your body will only use the protein it requires to build things; the rest becomes carbs.

Next, the sugars are used to supply the body's energy needs. Leftover sugars can be stored in the liver in a form called glycogen. There is also a minimal amount of glycogen stored in your muscle tissue. The glycogen store in your liver is enough energy to live on for a day or two.

When you go a few hours without eating anything, your blood sugar drops and glycogen is quickly pulled and used. If you haven't eaten anything all day, or if you ran a marathon this morning, your glycogen stores are probably running pretty low. If there is an extreme excess of sugars or proteins eaten, then your body is forced to manufacture more fats because your liver only has limited storage space.

Finally, the fats are taken from the bloodstream as well. As with protein, a certain amount of fats are needed each day for building purposes. After those needs are met, leftover fats are deposited into adipocytes. Unlike the glycogen stores, the fat reserves are almost unlimited. The adipocytes will grow bigger as more fat is deposited into them.

There are basic, logical reasons that fat has become the chosen energy store of our bodies. Fat stores are efficient. Within the chemical bonds of a gram of fat, there are nine calories. A gram of protein or a gram of carbohydrates only contains four calories. A gram of alcohol has seven calories, but the properties of alcohol allow it to travel easily throughout your body. It probably wouldn't ever stay put in your gut if your body decided to try and stash it there. Fat also requires fewer calories each day for maintenance than lean tissues, so that is another reason for its efficiency.

As far as digestion goes, the alcohol, vitamins, minerals, carbohydrates, fats, and proteins have been taken out of the chyme before it reaches the end of the intestines. The only thing left is any indigestible part of the original food and some bacteria from your colon. Portions of food that can't be digested are called fiber. They still play an important role in digestion even though they don't provide any calories. The fiber aids in overall movement and speeds up the digestive process by adding bulk. That's its purpose. And when it has served its purpose, our body...gets rid of it.

All in all, our bodies have a carefully executed strategy to glean the most possible calories from the food we eat and make the best use of them. Your body is programmed to save any extra energy as fat, which is why it sometimes seems hard to lose and easy to gain. Luckily, enough scientists have poked around our biology to find out ways to successfully lose weight. There are simple ways to get around the extremely energy-efficient methods of the human body.

CHAPTER 4

Calories Out vs. Calories In

So what IS the secret to weight loss? You may have listened to some "experts" on infomercials or read a few articles, and now you are completely confused. Should you eat only certain food groups? Eat only at certain times of day? Eat all raw foods instead of cooked? Avoid certain food combinations? Why are there so many diets out there? Why are there constantly new diets being created?

I'm going to let you in on a secret. Actually, it's not really very secret at all; it is common, accepted knowledge in the medical community. The National Institute of Health and the Center for Disease Control and all of the other big government-sponsored health research centers figured this one out years ago and moved on to alien autopsies. The secret to weight loss isn't a secret, but a fact: to lose weight you have to be using more calories than you are eating. This concept is typically referred to as "calories in versus calories out."

You can think of your entire day as a large calorie equation. If you were alive today, or at least for part of the day, you can make an equation. Your equation will include all of the things you ate or drank that include calories and all of the things that you or your body did to use up calories. Your personal equation might go something like this:

▶ + A bowl of cereal and oj for breakfast,

▶ - walking to your car,

▶ + doughnut at work,

▶ + two packets of sugar in your coffee,u

▶ - the energy to breathe and type while sitting at your computer,

▶ + a mid-afternoon Coke,

▶ - walking back to your car,

▶ - walking the dog,

▶ + fast-food dinner,

▶ - walking to your couch,

▶ - minus picking up the remote,

▶ + a midnight snack.

Now that was a very rough equation. Clearly, each day your body will use a certain amount of calories just to think, to circulate blood in your veins, and to breathe. This energy is required daily to stay alive (and, as you are probably aware, if you do not eat, you will not stay alive.) These are the types of calories that are necessary, but don't vary that much from day to day.

Try not to get too hung up on these "basic housekeeping" calories. They don't change much. They will always be there and be needed. The most significant factors in your equation are the "pluses" and "minuses" mentioned in the example equation. You can't control how many calories your body will use to maintain your body heat, but you CAN significantly control your food intake (pluses) and physical activity (minuses.) It is this balance between food eaten and activities done that is the secret key to weight loss. The equation doesn't lie, and you have the power to balance your own calorie equation.

If you can make any changes so that your personal equation results in a net loss each day, then your weight will go down. Changes might include things like eating less food total or switching a food with more calories for a different food with fewer calories. Changes might include things like adding a workout into your day. Changes might include just moving around more throughout the day, walking or riding your bike when you go somewhere, and regularly taking the stairs instead of the elevator.

If your personal daily equation comes out even at the end of the day, your weight will be maintained. This is likely to happen if you continue your current eating habits and current level of activity. It could also happen if you switch some factors in your equation, but you switch them for another factor with a similar calorie value. For example, you may change your doughnut for a candy bar. You are probably eating around the same amount of calories, so there is no net result. Another example would be if you changed the time you spent on the computer for an equal time playing videogames. Chances are that you would burn about the same amount of calories doing these two different activities. Change alone isn't enough; you must switch two foods or activities with different calorie values to see a change in body weight.

If you have changed some things in your equation for higher calorie factors, then you will see a net gain in your personal equation. That is, your weight will increase. To cause this, you may have changed something like walking with your dog. Maybe you walk him for less time than you used to, or maybe you passed the job off to your wife. This change will show up at the end of your calorie equation. Your net gain could also be a result of a change in your eating. Maybe the fast food place is having a special and so you have started eating a sundae in additional to your regular meal. Changes in your equation will be evident by your gaining or losing weight. Personal control of the equation is the only way for anyone to successfully lose weight.

If this is true, then why do so many people swear by the Atkin's diet or the grapefruit diet? The truth is that ALL diets make use of the "calories in versus calories out" concept, whether they explain it is those terms or not. Most diets work by making food more complicated or restricted, and thereby reducing your daily "pluses" in the equation. If all you can eat is meat, chances are you are soon going to be sick of it and just eat less overall. If the book says you can only eat a carb with a fruit, it's not because there is something magical about that combination, it's just that they are taking away your ability to eat fast-food combo meals, which is a heavy "plus" in the equation.

You can put actual numbers to the "calories in versus calories out" concept. A calorie is actually a measurement of energy, just like a watt or a kilojoule, etc. A calorie is equal to the amount of energy required to heat one kilogram of water one degree Celsius. The method originally used to measure the amount of calories in a food was by bomb calorimeter. Essentially, the food is put into a sturdy, closed container surrounded by water. When the food is burned, the increase in the water temperature is used to determine the calorie content. From these experiments, standard equations were developed so that today food manufacturers can estimate the calorie content of their foods just by knowing their percentage of protein, fat, carbohydrate, and alcohol.

Just as foods contain predictable amounts of calories, so too does the body use energy in a predictable way. Extra calories from days of net gain in your personal calorie equation are deposited in adipocytes, or fat cells. A pound of body fat from any body anywhere in the world will contain 3,500 calories' worth of energy. That is why I can predict that if you eat an extra bowl of ice cream that contains about 200 calories tonight after dinner, and you continue to do this daily without changing any other aspect of your equation, you will have gained one pound by day eighteen. If you don't believe me, try it. Or better yet, try working your equation the opposite way: Starting today, switch your daily regular 20 oz. Cherry Coke for a glass of water. At approx. 266 calories per Coke, you will lose one pound in about fourteen days.

Because it takes 3500 calories to lose one pound, this is not something that can be done quickly. 3500 is probably a lot more calories than you even need for a whole day. And even if you don't eat for a day or two (something that doesn't sound healthy or fun), your body does not just give you a pound. For the couple of days that you don't eat, your body will run on its glycogen store in your liver. That's what it's there for. Then, if you continue to not eat or under eat, you body will start getting rid of some muscles that you have. They take a lot of calories each day, and you're not eating, so your body has no choice. The loss of muscles plus the slowing down of a few body functions (try figuring out a hard problem at work if you're not eating; it's going to be rough) takes your total basal metabolism down a notch. For our purposes, "a notch" is about ten percent. Then, if you begin eating like a normal person again, you need even less calories per day and more of what you eat goes in the "extra" storage pile. Yikes.

So an all-out battle on your personal calorie equation isn't going to work in your favor. It will probably make you mad and make you realize that your body is, in fact, a true survivor. It might even explain why you made it out of the jungle and some of your early ancestors did not.

Clearly, a more subtle approach is required. If your body doesn't know that this is a fight, it will give up the fat stores much more easily than if you ambush it head-on. In other words, you have to make changes, but avoid tripping up any alarms. The best way to do this is to only eliminate a moderate amount of calories each day. The National Heart, Lung, and Blood Institute recommends that people try not to lose more than one or two pounds of weight each week maximum. Those who lose at this slow, healthy rate have been shown to be successful with their weight loss and to keep the weight off in the long-term, and that is most likely what you are aiming to do yourself. One to two pounds is just about the right sneaky amount to secret away per week.

If you are losing one pound a week, that means that each day you are eating 500 calories less, exercising 500 calories more, or eating 250 calories less and also exercising 250 calories more. That is actually a fairly significant lifestyle change. Consider that a two hundred pound man who walks for an hour at a rate of seventeen minutes per mile burns about 450 calories total. So if our two hundred pound man starts today and walks for an hour every day at this pace (assuming he is in good enough shape not to injure himself with this routine), and continues to eat the same way, it will take just over a week to lose one pound.

If he doesn't know much about weight loss, he might feel like he is doing a whole lot of work with not much of a result to show for it. He has probably seen a lot of "lose thirty pounds in thirty days" weight-loss advertising around town and wonders why he isn't doing even better, since he's trying to do it the healthy way. The thing is that the poor guy is doing it the right way; he's just getting frustrated because he has unrealistic expectations about what his body can physically do. It's not realistic for someone to lose much more than fifty pounds in one year. The good news is that he is successfully manipulating his personal calorie equation and getting the results that he wants.

The "3500 calories per pound" concept is easy enough to grasp, but how do you know what figure you need to take those 250-500 daily calories off of? You must create your daily calorie deficit by subtracting these calories from the total amount needed to maintain your current level of activity and your body at its current size.

There are several different equations that can be used if you want to estimate your daily calorie needs. These equations range from very, very specific to general rule-of-thumb estimates. On the specific end are the equations used by registered dietitians working in the Intensive Care Unit to cal-

culate intravenous feedings for victims of trauma. If they
calculate calorie requirements too low, the patient doesn't
optimize recovery, and if they estimate the calorie requirements to be too high, they can send the patient into multiple
system organ failure. Because of the sensitivity of the situation, equations such as these factor in things like total
percentage of the body covered in burns and whether any
limbs are missing, all things that could potentially cause in-
accurate calorie calculations.

It's unlikely that you need to know with such certitude what
your exact daily calorie needs are. A healthy body is much
more flexible. On the other end of the spectrum of calorie estimation, there are national recommendations based on
age group and gender. For example, all relatively sedentary
males between the ages of twenty-one and forty are estimated
to need 2,400 calories a day.

For someone interested in a somewhat personalized calcu-
lation that falls short of the specificity of intensive medical
care, an equation in the "middle ground" is the best option.
First decide which group your daily lifestyle falls into: sedentary, moderately active, or heavy activity. Resist the urge to
calculate according to the lifestyle you wish you were living,
the lifestyle you lived ten years ago, or the lifestyle that you
plan to start up here in a couple of days.

Typically "sedentary" is considered to be a lifestyle that includes less than a half hour of activity each day. If you
basically just get up, go to work where you sit for the ma-

jority of the day, and come home, then you are considered sedentary. It sounds unpleasant, but it is true.

A moderately active person might have the same habits as the first person, except they also take thirty to sixty minutes each afternoon to go walking at a brisk pace. Someone else might not do any walking or other exercise, but they work full time and are on their feet all day. If you are doing at least a half hour of an aerobic activity, then you qualify as moderately active. And any activity that gets your heart rate up and gets you to the point where you are starting to sweat can be counted as aerobic; it doesn't have to be on a machine at the gym. You body sure doesn't know the difference.

Finally, the designation "heavy activity" is reserved for the all-out athlete. If you are currently in boot camp or practice at least an hour a day with your hockey/soccer/basketball team, then this is you. If you are not quite sure if you belong in the "heavy activity" group or the "moderately active" group, you are moderately active. People who do heavy activity do it on purpose. They know that they are doing heavy activity.

The next step to complete before using the equation is to convert your weight from pounds to kilograms. If you are an American that knows what you weigh in kilograms, good for you! If you are like the other 98% of Americans, you will need to divide your weight in pounds by 2.2.

Now you can begin the calorie calculations. If you determined yourself to be sedentary, you will need about 25-30 calories per kilogram of body weight. Multiply 25 by your weight in kilograms and you are good to go. Hold this subtotal until the next step. Moderately active individuals need about 35 calories per kilogram of body weight. And finally, the star athletes are looking at about 40 calories per kilogram.

There is one more step to figure out your total daily calorie needs. It is an adjustment for age, since basal metabolism slows down over time. Take the total that you came up with in the last step and subtract 100 calories for every decade that you have lived past thirty years. (Sorry, it's not age discrimination, just biological truth.)

You now have a decent approximation of your daily calorie needs. If you eat this many calories each day and maintain your current activity level, your weight should stay exactly the same (until you are ten years older, when you may have to shave off another 100 calories to maintain.)

The lucky thing is that the actual numerical calculations are unnecessary for the average person trying to lose weight. In your body there is a large built-in response system: if you gain weight, it is too many calories. If you maintain, then you are right on target, and if you lose, well, hopefully that's because you were trying to.

So you're probably thinking that this really doesn't sound

too bad. If your body religiously follows this equation, and you've got a calculator, you can beat it at its own game. Which is definitely true. But there is a catch. If you lose one pound from fourteen days of Coke-free lunches, you cannot go back to the Coke from day fifteen through the rest of your life and expect to keep that pound off. It won't work. Calories in versus calories out is applicable for your entire lifespan.

CHAPTER 5

How to Burn Calories

Previous chapters have explained that essentially the body burns calories whenever it is forced to move, a process commonly called "exercising." Energy is also used for body processes, specifically powering electrical impulses in your nervous system and ion concentration pumps to keep you hydrated.

Calories that are burned each day can also be divided into four different subcategories (in order of calories burned from most to least): basal metabolism, physical activity, the thermic effect of food, and Non-Exercise Activity Thermogenesis. The last two are most likely unfamiliar. Except for nutrition researchers on lunch break, there are not many people who sit around and talk about these concepts!

Most of the calories burned by the body each day are included in the 'calories required for basal metabolism. Your basal metabolism is a very bare bones minimum that your body needs to survive. If you want to live on just your basal metabolic calories, your body isn't going to give you any fancy extras like warming you up if the room is chilly. You won't get any body movement included in the deal either. And there is definitely no digestion processes included. The basal metabolism will only cover you sitting in a comfortably heated room, awake but motionless, not thinking too hard, and hungry. Surprisingly, the majority of your calories each day go to funding your basal metabolism.

Metabolism is a current buzzword in society. Even little kids will say things like, "oh, it's just my bad metabolism," without knowing what it really means. They just heard their moms say it before. Incidentally, their moms probably don't know what it really means either. Most people will tell you that it has something to do with weight loss. It's the magic something extra that everyone needs. You probably hear a lot about "ways to boost your metabolism" and special things you can do to maximize your metabolism. Interestingly, a lot of the supposed metabolism boosting methods involve the public having to purchase an untested supplement that was probably manufactured somewhere where no one knows what goes in those pills. Actually, that place could be the U.S. The federal government currently does not test or approve herbal or weight loss supplements the way it does with drugs. Sometimes things do eventually get pulled off of the shelves and banned, but only because people started dying from taking the product! Be very wary of anyone who claims to be able to change your body's metabolism.

Each individual person will not experience much day-to-day change in basal metabolism. There are some metabolism-changing factors that can occur over time, but they are minimal. However, when comparing the basal metabolic rates of different people, there can be differences of up to 25 or 30% These discrepancies can be attributed to a few factors.

First of all, some people have more body surface than other people. More heat is lost in people with more body surface area, so their metabolisms are higher, that is, they require slightly more calories each day to maintain themselves. It's like how kids like to eat soup out of shallower bowls so that it isn't as hot and they can eat it faster without burning their tongues. A shallow bowl spreads the soup out so that there is more surface area touching the air and letting off heat. In the soup situation, the additional surface area is a good thing, but as far as bodies go, it makes it tougher to survive. Your body keeps churning out the energy, trying to keep you at 98.6 degrees, but if you're tall and gangly, you are wasting a lot of the heat once it's produced. A short and stocky body build is the most energy-efficient and will require a lower basal metabolism to keep it going.

The next factor determining your basal metabolism is more transitory than your total body surface area, but it is also related to body temperature. If maintaining yourself at a healthy 98.6 degrees Fahrenheit takes X calories, getting your body temperature up to a toasty 100.0 degrees even is going to take X + a few more. So if you get the flu and run a fever for several days, your basal metabolism is going to go up as your body shovels some more coal on the fire. Calorie-wise, it is a little more expensive than a healthy body temperature, but overall it can be a good investment for your body. It is basically a military maneuver against internal invaders. The idea is that your body will raise its own temperature high enough that it might be able to kill the bacteria or virus that is attacking it. It is a fine line to tread, though. If the fever goes past a certain temperature, your own body proteins begin to be cooked and are no longer able to perform their duties. Hopefully that never happens to you, no matter how many calories you could potentially spend in the process!

The next factor that influences your daily basal metabolism is your age. Kids are not going to be included in this summary, because their bodies are using lots of energy for other things like growing and fighting off the germs that they picked up while riding the bus home from school. Plus, they burn a ton of calories because they never actually sit down and stop twitching. Among the adult set, young adults are the highest calorie burners with the highest metabolisms. They tend to have more muscle mass, which helps, and their bodies are in the peak functioning years.

Metabolism does slowly decline as a person ages. It usually turns out to be about a 2% decline every ten years after you turn thirty. It's really not a huge change. If you used to be able to eat 2,400 calories a day, which, according to Uncle Sam is most sedentary young adult males, then at age forty you would officially lose 48 of those calories. That's like half of a low-fat yogurt cup or four and a half less potato chips each day. Many adults do feel a drastic change in their ability to maintain their weight after they enter middle age. It is much more likely the fault of their changing lifestyle than their dropping metabolism. Somehow, there is a magic age where the kids don't need chased around every day and you also start making a little more money than you used to. Usually this translates into more going out to eat and more paying other, younger, more poor-and-desperate people to do your manual labor for you. So don't blame your metabolism.

If there truly is something biological at fault for your difficulty with losing weight, it may be your thyroid. Thyroid issues are very well known causes of metabolism problems. If you go to your doctor complaining about losing weight uncontrollably or about not being able to lose weight no matter how many miles you walk, one of the first things he or she will check will be your thyroid.

The thyroid is in charge of releasing certain hormones that control your metabolism into your bloodstream. Most people's bodies release just the right amount, the "right amount" being determined by all of the factors governing how much energy your body needs to maintain. If sickness, surgery, or radiation treatment damages your thyroid, it could under- or over-release the thyroid hormones. An excess of thyroid hormones is called hyperthyroidism, and this condition will speed up your metabolism. If you have hyperthyroidism, you will probably be losing weight, not able to sleep, and feeling pretty edgy.

Hypothyroidism is the opposite problem, and it is much more common. In this case, your thyroid isn't giving off enough hormones to keep your metabolism going at full speed, so weight loss is more difficult. People with hypothyroidism typically feel tired as well. At this point, you may be tempted to self-diagnose, but in reality you need a blood test from your doctor to know for sure. People with a lack of thyroid hormones have to take artificial hormones in order to bring their bodies up to speed.

The final factor involved in determining a person's metabolism is pretty much the only one that can be controlled. Efforts to change your body surface area or give yourself a fever or hyperthyroidism would be pretty ridiculous. You're also probably not going to find a way to un-age ten years to get your 2% back. However, your nutritional state is something that you have control over.

The body has some amount of discretion in how efficient it should be with its calories. If it has been a normal month or so and it has been fed regularly, it will use the higher end of the possibility. There is really no reason for it to be concerned. However, if there are any signs of danger of food shortage, your body can immediately become even more conservative with calorie use. Your body doesn't know if there is a famine going on in the outside world when you don't eat regularly or don't eat enough. It just knows that it hasn't been getting enough, so it's time to pull back. You may have heard people tell you not to diet too much or you might " put your body into starvation mode." This is exactly what they are talking about!

Your body is generally as efficient as possible, so there is not a large portion of calories to cut back on. If a person is in a poor nutritional state (aka they aren't eating enough), then their basal metabolism will be reduced by about 150-300 calories per day. It's not huge, but it is significant. To avoid this problem, don't skip meals or try to cut out more than 500 calories or so each day. Unfortunately, your nutritional state is one of the few ways that you can change your metabolism, and it is only possible to make a negative change. Overeating doesn't make your body burn extra calories each day in your basal metabolism.

That's a lot of metabolism talk, but the basal metabolism is only the first (and biggest) of four ways that the body burns calories every day. Next in line are the calories needed for physical activity. An active person might increase their calorie needs to 25% or even 40% of their metabolic needs. An inactive person could stay much closer just needed their basal metabolic calories each day. Someone who was bedridden, for example, wouldn't need many physical activity calories at all. If this person was previously active and was forced to rest due to illness or injury, they may find it difficult to eat any differently than they used to when they were feeling good. Because of this difference in calories used and eaten, it is pretty easy to gain weight while on bed rest.

Physical activity is the factor that varies the most widely between individuals. Whereas the basal metabolism differs slightly due to an individual's size, body temperature, age and nutritional state, physical activity runs the full gamut. On one end, there are people on bed rest who can move very little throughout the day. On the other extreme, there are people who train for things like ultra marathons. (An ultra marathon is much longer than "just" a marathon. I wonder who came up with that brilliant idea.)

The third use of calories by the body each day is for something called "the Thermic Effect of Food." It is usually referred to as just TEF, probably since so many people already know what it means. The Thermic Effect of Food is a much less significant portion of the total calories than either the basal metabolism or physical activity. It basically means the amount of calories used to digest food.

Digestion is a complicated process that isn't "free," caloriewise. The chewing of the food, the stomach-juice making, the nutrient absorption process, and the transport of the carbohydrates, fats, and proteins around to their places in the body isn't cheap. However, clearly there is a net gain during the eating process, or eating wouldn't be a productive activity for your body! Really you only lose a relatively small percentage of the total calories contained in the food to the action of digestion. The Thermic Effect of Food takes off about 5% to 10% of the total calorie value of the food you are eating.

This percentage does not differ in regards to digestion. Digestion is digestion, and it has happened pretty predictably for thousands of years. The difference comes because of the calorie value of the foods being digested. A high calorie food goes through the same digestive process as a low calorie food. Therefore, when a stomach is full of fast food and candy (which are very calorie-dense foods), your body takes off the same flat fee for digestion. If you have to digest a stomach full of fruits and vegetables (which are not very calorie-dense foods), your body takes off the same digestion fee, but gains less calories from the food. So with less calorie dense foods, the percentage of those calories used for digestion is higher.

It is the principal of the Thermic Effect of Food that is sometimes used to explain the need for dieters to eat a lot of celery. The idea is that celery has few calories, but still needs to be digested if you eat it. So theoretically, by eating a lot of celery each day, you could actually use up more calories by eating! It sounds like a really good idea, until you realize that the calories you burn are minimal. Plus you have to continuously eat a ton of celery; some dieters recommend about three bunches per day! No matter how much you like celery, you will be force-feeding yourself after a day on this plan.

The fourth and final way that your body uses calories each day is called "Non-Exercise Activity Thermogenesis." Like all really good scientific terms, it has a great acronym you can use instead: NEAT. Non-Exercise Activity Thermogenesis is basically just a fancy term that means you can't sit still. Look at the term more closely; it is saying that it includes all calorie-burning activities that aren't exercise.

Essentially, this includes nervous habits, ticks, and general restlessness. People who fidget more burn more calories by way of NEAT.

Non-Exercise Activity Thermogenesis was not on the list of "ways to burn calories" a few years ago. It is a fairly recent (and accidental) discovery. While doing some studies, nutritional researchers noticed that some people don't seem to gain weight even if they eat more calories than they need. They reasoned that these people had to be burning off these extra calories somehow. After more careful observation and more studies, they realized that the people who maintained their weight were the fidgeters in the group. Apparently, some people, when overfed, are a lot more antsy and their movement allows them to burn off the extra calories that they have eaten. A good way to remember this concept is to think of a kid who just ate too much candy. Typically there is a lot of stray movement and twitching that comes into play. That's Non-Exercise Activity Thermogenesis.

Unfortunately, information about NEAT probably isn't very helpful to anyone except nutrition researchers (and parents who want to know why their kids do what they do.) If you already fidget, that's fine; it burns calories. If you don't fidget, then it is unlikely that you would spontaneously start to control your weight.

The moral of this chapter is that, although your body burns calories in a few different ways, the only one that you have any control over and is significant enough to make a difference is physical activity. That is why it is so important to be physically active to lose weight. It is the best way, and virtually the only way to burn extra calories each day.

In order for physical activity to be effective for weight loss, it needs to be consistent over time. Consistency means you do it every day, or every other day. Say you feel inspired tomorrow and decide that, after fourteen years of sitting, you are going to make a change. So you go chop firewood for four hours and then attempt to play backyard football with your nephews until the sun goes down. This is how to get injured, not how to lose weight. Start slow, start at your current fitness level and work up to harder activities. Whatever activity you choose needs to be done consistently. Do it all or most days of the week year-round to get maximum fitness and weight loss benefits.

CHAPTER 6

How to Reduce Intake of Calories

After analyzing your personal calorie equation in detail, you may have come to the conclusion that you need to reduce your intake of calories to help you to lose weight. There are, of course, many, many ways to go about that. Some of them may be objectively better ideas, as far as health status is concerned. Some of them might be better ideas for you personally, being more feasible options in your lifestyle. Careful consideration at the beginning of the weight loss process can help you to identify the techniques for reducing calories that are going to help you to be the most successful in the long run.

"How do I reduce my intake of calories?" It is a deceptively simple question. It's a question that millions of people have asked themselves and their doctors. The very short answer to this question is "eat less food." However, the short answer probably hasn't helped many individuals to successfully lose weight. The reason this is such an in-depth topic is that you know that you want the outcome to be a reduction in calories, but you don't know how to go about doing this. Knowing to eat less and being able to successfully eat less over a long time period are two very different things.

The long answer to the question of how to reduce consumption of calories is much longer than this book. It may not even be possible to document all of the ways that anyone has ever tried to cut calories from their diet. Each person is very individual and different solutions may work for some people and not others. "Working" or "not working" refers to whether or not a person can reasonably manage to adhere to the technique. If any of these methods are done accurately , it will definitely work in the sense that it will help you to lose weight. It has to work because it follows the "calories in versus calories out" rule, just like everything else.

One of the most obvious and basic approaches to reducing your daily calorie intake is called "portion control." This is as close as it gets to the short answer of "just eat less." The term "portion" refers to the amount of a food that is eaten at one time. It can be different every time you eat a food. Maybe for dinner last night you ate a portion of steak that was 8 oz. Next week you might have a different portion, like a 10 oz. portion. If you eat just a couple of bites of steak from someone else's plate, then that is a much smaller portion, maybe even a fraction of an ounce.

In nutrition terminology, portions are very different than servings, but the two words are often confused in general conversation. A serving is a set amount of a given food. There are official serving sizes for any food that you would want to eat. The government sets these serving sizes and they are used to influence manufacturers' food labeling. For example, a serving size of ice cream is one half cup. That is standard. Every brand of ice cream in the aisle has the same serving size on its label. This standard serving size allows you to easily compare the nutrition facts between different flavors and brands of ice cream.

The serving sizes are not always quite so uniform, though. For some products there is a range that is acceptable for the serving size. Usually the expensive, bad-for-you crackers list their serving size to be four crackers, whereas the regular saltines might give you five crackers in one serving.

If you were to eat one whole sleeve of crackers in a sitting, this is your portion. The serving size is still four crackers; that does not change. Portions are made at your discretion. Slightly larger portions give you more calories in your diet. Portion control means that you are attempting to restrict your portions of food to a reasonable level. A good goal is the original serving size. If you typically put about a cup and a half of ice cream in your bowl, you may try limiting yourself to just the one half cup of ice cream. You can still have crackers with your soup, but try eating just five. You can use the serving size on the nutrition facts label on food packages to give you a good idea for a portion size of that food.

Most people find that portion control is an adjustment at first, but later on it becomes a very natural for them. Our minds get used to seeing similar amounts of food in front of us and come to expect it. If you currently eat half of a large bag of chips in one sitting, a small handful probably seems like a far-off dream. Just work your portions down bit by bit over time, and rest assured that you will get used to it eventually.

Luckily, scientists have done multiple studies on the human brain in regards to how it sees food and portion sizes. These studies have resulted in several useful pieces of information for the average dieter. First of all, we humans tend to eat what is put in front of us. If there is more available, we tend to eat more overall. For example, if you could give three different people various amounts of pretzels and tell them to eat whatever they want and stop when they are full. Suppose you gave one person a cup of pretzels, the second person two cups of pretzels, and the third person three cups of pretzels. The first person might eat half a cup of pretzels or so. The second person would probably eat more than the first. Chances are that the third person would eat the most of all, since more total was available. We tend to judge food relative to its surroundings, not by its own quantity. The take-home message here is to figure out what a reasonable portion of food is and put that on your plate or in your bowl or cup. Then put the rest away. You will most likely eat more overall if you eat out of the package. At home, take out a handful of pretzels and put them in a bowl to eat. Don't sit down with the whole bag of pretzels; you will most likely eat more without even realizing it.

Another thing to keep in mind is the size of plates and silverware that you eat with at home. Plates with larger diameters have become more common in the past few years. People used to eat off of much smaller plates. Your "medium-sized" plates are probably closer in size to the dinner plates your parents ate from when they were your age. Again, the brain judges the relative size of the food portion, not the absolute size. A half-cup of mashed potatoes looks decent on a small plate, but on a larger plate, it looks puny.

This concept was well illustrated by one study that provided ice cream at a faculty meeting with nutrition professors and researchers. This was done on two different days, once with a bigger ice cream scoop and bowls, and on another day with a smaller ice cream scoop and bowls. These subjects were not "ordinary" people; they were experts in the field of nutrition and weight! They also knew that it was a study, because the researchers weighed the bowl of ice cream that each person served themselves before they could start eating. Even with all of these advantages, the professors still served themselves significantly larger portions when they were working with the large ice cream scoop and large bowl.

Buying some smaller plates, glasses, bowls, and silverware for everyday use will make it much easier for you to cut your portion sizes. Eating a sundae that is completely filling a small dessert bowl is more satisfying than eating what looks like a dollop of ice cream out of an oversized mixing bowl. Do yourself a favor and work that optical illusion for your benefit!

Portion control is a very helpful tool to help reduce the overall calories that you eat each day. It also has the advantage that you do not have to change the types of foods that you eat each day at all. You can eat what you would normally eat for breakfast, lunch, dinner, and snacks, but in a smaller portion, and still lose weight. If you already eat a reasonably well-rounded diet, but need to lose weight, working on reducing your portions is probably a great place for you to start.

Another popular technique for reducing the amount of calories that are eaten in a day is sometimes called "mindful eating." It is based on the idea that a person cannot even judge his or her own hunger and fullness cues if distracted by other activities during mealtimes. To become a more mindful eater, you have to only do one thing while eating: eat! This concept can be surprisingly difficult for people who are already accustomed to eating and driving, eating and working, and eating and watching television. It might even be interesting to remember what sitting down to a meal by itself really feels like.

If this approach sounds woefully foreign to your current eating habits, you can start with just one mindful meal per week or so. You can get used to the feeling gradually. To make your meal, be sure to put the food on plates; don't eat it out of the packages. Try to really taste what your food tastes like and enjoy the smell and texture and everything that comes with eating. Make the eating atmosphere comfortable. Invite some people that you like to eat with you if you want. Eating and enjoying the company should be the only activities going on. Typically, people eat more slowly when they are in an enjoyable location, and they eat less overall than when they cram whatever they can find in their mouths in ten minutes while they are watching television.

The lack of distractions present during mealtimes helps a person to be more aware of their body signals. If you are not thinking about if you are satisfied, most likely you will keep eating until you realize that you most certainly are full. Probably a little too full, actually. However, if you have been paying attention, you are more likely to identify that point in time when it would be good to stop.

Biological hunger signals actually provide the basis for another popular method for reducing calorie intake. From the moment that you begin to eat something, it takes the body approximately twenty minutes to be able to sense that you have eaten something. That is considerable lag time for a body that seems so efficient in so many ways, but that's how long it takes. Now think about how much food you could eat in twenty minutes, especially if you were really hungry. The average person could probably eat at least one large pizza. The problem with that is that after you have eaten is when you will feel the effects of your hunger cues, and then it is too late.

This is a fantastic argument for eating more slowly in general. People typically do eat more slowly if they are paying attention to and enjoying their food. In a nice restaurant, people eat more slowly. This is an advantage, because you have the chance to truly judge when you are full.

Besides eating more slowly, there is another way to take advantage of the fact that all food takes about twenty minutes to register with your brain. People who prefer this method reason that the whole problem with the twenty minutes is that when people are really hungry, they eat really quickly. So instead of forcing themselves to eat more slowly, they will try to avoid getting hungry. How can you do that? By having a very regular eating schedule. If you break up your bigger meals into a series of smaller meals throughout the day, say six meals instead of three, then you don't get those time gaps when your stomach starts to growl. One caveat is that you have to always have food around to be able to maintain your continuous eating pattern. This could be difficult if there is no refrigerator where you work, or if your schedule is inflexible. Another possible caveat is that it may be difficult to remember to eat smaller meals. Even though you are eating more times per day, the goal is to lose weight, so you should be eating less food overall.

Despite the possible caveats for the "small meals" trick, a lot of people really find it to be a good method since they tend to be able to both lose weight and feel full all day, which are two things not traditionally associated with each other. There is also the possibility of doing your own sort of mix between a typical diet and a six-meals-per-day plan. For example, instead of six little meals, you could try eating three light meals a day and two snacks, one in the morning and one in the afternoon. This hybrid can be pretty potent as well as be more compatible with a busy schedule..

Avoiding hunger even though you are cutting calories is a pretty popular idea, and there are other ways to achieve this without spreading out your eating schedule. For example, you can attempt to increase the volume of the food in your stomach while decreasing the total calorie amount of the food. This idea comes from a concept called "stomach distention." Scientists have spent a lot of time trying to identify what exactly it is that triggers our bodies to signal that we are full. One of the factors identified was stomach distention, or the expanding of your stomach,. Your stomach is stretchable and it seems that once it has stretched to a certain degree, that can trigger you to fell satisfied and not want to eat any more. So the trick is to get your stomach to expand by filling it with low-calorie foods. Then you won't have eaten that many of your total daily calories, but you won't be too hungry either.

There are several food possibilities for increasing the total volume of the food that you eat. The most significant of these is fiber. Fiber is the non-digestible part of many plant foods that we eat. The best sources of fiber are fruits, vegetables, legumes (like beans), and whole grain bread products. You can make simple changes such as eating an orange instead of drinking orange juice. Orange juice is just an orange without the fiber! Adding more of fiber-rich foods to your diet will help you to increase your overall food volume, but simultaneously reduce the total calories consumed. It's actually pretty sneaky.

Water can be used in the same way to increase food volume. Studies have shown that the most effective way to decrease your hunger with water is not to drink more water (although that certainly does help some people), but to eat more watery foods. For example, if you eat a bowl of soup before a meal, chances are that you will eat less at the meal because you have already filled yourself up on the soup.

Of course, for a soup to be used for this purpose, it has to be fairly low-calorie. That automatically rules out all of the cream-based and cheese-based soups. A low-calorie, high volume soup would be broth based and light. Think of something like vegetable soup, chicken soup, or a bean soup. If you are in doubt whether a soup is low-calorie or not, check the label or make it at home so that you can see what goes into it. If it is soup from a restaurant, it probably isn't low-calorie no matter what type of soup it is. Restaurants have a really bad habit of putting a lot of extra fat into everything, even when nobody can really taste the difference. So to best take advantage of the idea of increasing your food volume, start your meals with light soups, vegetables, and/or fruits.

Liquid calories in the form of soup can be a good thing, but other caloric liquids can really be bad news in your quest to reduce your calorie intake. You drink liquid calories when you have coffee with creamer and sugar, regular soda, chocolate milk, juice, Kool-Aid, etc. All of these drinks aren't necessarily bad: chocolate milk can be a good way to get in your servings of dairy, and 100% fruit juice does still count as fruit. The thing is that there are still a lot of calories in these beverages, and the calories are surprisingly easy to consume when in liquid form. To go back to the orange juice example, you probably don't usually eat six or seven oranges in one sitting, but a large glass of orange juice isn't so strange. That's because liquid calories are very stealthy. They seem to somehow avoid triggering any "fullness" clues in the body, so they are used for energy, but you don't end up feeling any fuller.

One particular researcher noticed that something fishy was going on with the liquid calories. To test this theory, he did a study with jellybeans and regular soda. Jellybeans and soda are both essentially pure sugar, just in different forms. The study consisted of two groups. One group got the jellybeans every day and the other group got soda. The amount of calories in the jellybeans was the same as the amount of calories in the portion of soda. The subjects were allowed to eat whatever else that they wanted throughout the day. The interesting result was that the jellybean group tended to eat less other foods when they ate the jellybeans. They must have felt fuller and so it was natural for them to eat less of something else throughout the day. This wasn't the case with the soda group. They ate exactly the same amount of food that they usually did, but also drank the soda. So the soda group ended up having several hundred more calories each day without even noticing the difference.

Some scientists speculate that maybe our bodies weren't set up to be able to read liquid calories. Caloric beverages are a somewhat recent invention, or at least we certainly drink a lot more calories than people used to. Humans originally had only water after they were weaned.

For many people trying to lose weight these days, portion control and avoiding liquid calories go hand-in-hand. An 8 oz. cup of milk, soda, or juice is pretty reasonable, but a gas station fountain drink can have half of the calories that you need for the whole day! If you drink that much soda and still eat as you normally do, you could gain two pounds in one week. If you currently drink soda or certain creamy coffee beverages daily, cutting those out or replacing them with a non-caloric beverage could be the only change that you need to make to lose weight.

Portion control, mindful eating, increasing food volume, and avoiding liquid calories are some of the most common ways that people successfully reduce their intake of calories. Only you know what will be the most successful approach for you. Maybe it will be one of these approaches. Maybe it will be a combination of several different ideas. Maybe you even have a few other ideas in mind. Whatever plan you come up with, remember that you need to do it consistently over the long-term to see results. Pick something and stick with it and you will be successful!

CHAPTER 7

How to Keep Track of your Weight

Once you begin making changes in your personal calorie equation, you will begin to lose weight. At this point, you will probably want to find some way to gauge your loss. Are you losing at the ideal one-half to two pounds per week? More? Less? After you have lost weight to the point that you feel satisfied, how do you plan to maintain that weight? It's a good question to consider, and there are many ways to keep track of your weight.

At first thought, scales are the most obvious method used for tracking weight. That's definitely what they are designed to do, and they may be your preferred method. Some people like to weigh themselves every day, but that is probably excessive. Weighing yourself every day can put undue focus on the weight loss process. It's healthy to lose weight if you need to, but it's not healthy to be obsessed with the process.

Another drawback to daily weighing is that it makes the process feel ridiculously slow. If you are losing at a good healthy rate of one pound a week, then by weighing yourself daily you could see drops in increments of 1/7 of a pound. Chances are that your scale isn't that precise, so to you it will look like the scale is not moving. That's setting yourself up for frustration.

Another good thing to keep in mind is that your body weight can vary up to four pounds during the course of one day, depending on the time of day, your level of hydration, when you've eaten, etc. If you weigh yourself every day, it might seem like you are just jumping up and down a pound or two. Such fluctuations are normal and don't mean that you have really gained or lost any body fat, but they can really mess with your psyche. Weighing yourself once a week is plenty. Less than that is probably even better.

Scales are the classic, but not the only way to measure weight loss. There are possibly as many different ways to keep track of weight as there are people trying to lose weight. Think about how you can tell when you have lost or gained weight. There are little clues all over that may be unique to your body. A popular measure is the way that a particular article of clothing fits you over time. There may be a particular pair of pants that only fit you when you are in shape. Maybe there is a shirt that doesn't ever look good when you gain weight. As long as your article of clothing doesn't shrink in the laundry or stretch out over time, it can be a handy weight measurement tool.

Another good article of clothing that can be used to measure your weight loss with is a frequently worn belt. Your weight loss goals could be in belt holes instead of pounds. As you use different holes, you know that you must be losing weight around your middle. Another good reason to measure your weight this way is that weight loss around the middle of the body is more beneficial in terms of health.

There are typically two types of body weight patterns: the "apple" and the "pear." A pear-shaped body is one that gains weight more heavily on the bottom half. Pear- shaped people tend to have heavier thighs and legs and backsides, whereas they have smaller upper halves. An apple-shaped body is one that gains weight around the middle. Apple-shaped people gain their weight in their stomachs and chests. Overall, there are more women who are pear-shaped and more men who are apple-shaped. However, there are plenty of men who are pears and women who are apples.

The only reason this distinction between body shapes is important is that apple-shaped people tend to have higher risk for heart disease. Gaining weight around the middle seems to be more dangerous than gaining weight on the thighs. Because of this additional risk, monitoring weight by some measurement of middle body fat is a good idea. If you wear the same belt more or less daily, this may be the perfect measurement tool for you.

For people who infrequently wear belts, or who several different belts over the course of the week, a better option might be a tape measure. Knowing the measurement of your waist/stomach in inches is just as helpful, even though it is not quite as convenient as the belt trick. If using a tape measure to measure the widest part around your midsection, an important standard to remember is that a measurement of less than 40 inches is ideal. If your waist at the thickest point is more than 40 inches, it puts you at additional risk for heart disease. (This is just the numerical version of the apple-shaped/ pear-shaped test.)

Another advantage of using a tape measure instead of a belt is that more areas of the body can be assessed aside from the waist. Popular possibilities for other body areas to measure include thighs, hips, legs, calves, arms, and chest. This can give a much more comprehensive view of body changes over time.

If you have been working out regularly, and especially if your workouts include weight training, a tape measure could be the ideal measurement technique for you. Muscle tissue is more compact than fat tissue. That means that if you have five pounds of muscle, it will take up less space than if you have five pounds of fat. However, if you weigh yourself on a scale, there is no way to tell if you have traded in five pounds of fat for five pounds of muscle. If you are simultaneously losing body fat and gaining muscle, then you could theoretically even stay exactly the same weight.

Obviously, if you are becoming more fit and muscular, that is a healthy change, even if the scale doesn't show the difference. This is another reason for using a tape measure. If a person loses five pounds of fat and simultaneously gains five pounds of muscle, the scale won't show the difference, but the tape measure will. Being more compact, the more muscular person will measure less inches around the waist, legs, etc.

Just like measuring inches, measuring percent body fat gives more information about the composition of the body of the subject. However, percent body fat is a direct measure of body composition, whereas inches are an indirect measure of body composition. What is the point of knowing your body composition? The human body is made up of many different types of tissues that are classified into two main groups: the adipose tissue and everything else. These are also called fat tissues and lean tissues. Lean tissues include many different things like internal organs, muscles, and bones. Ideally, men have about 20% or less body fat and women have 30% or less of their bodies as body fat. Women have significantly more body fat because their bodies have to stockpile additional calories in order to be able to reproduce in times of famine. Men do not require this additional store, plus they generally have more muscle tissue, and so that increases their percentage of lean tissue.

Measurements of body composition are an ideal method for judging if someone is at a healthy body weight. It makes even more sense than weighing someone, because it takes into account different bone structures and different body builds.

The most accurate method for determining body composition is underwater weighing. As the name of the method
implies, the person being assessed is actually put into a tank
of water for the weighing process, wearing only a bathing
suit, if anything. When ready, the person being weighed
goes under the water in the tank (usually there are bars to
hold on to help him or her be completely submerged) and
exhales to blow out as much air from the lungs as possible.
A machine measures the total buoyancy of the body to determine the body composition. This is possible because fat
tissue floats and lean tissue does not. The percentages of fat
and lean tissues can be calculated by the body's tendency to
float.

One caveat is that the air in the lungs also floats. For this
reason, the subject to be weighed must exhale as completely
as possible. Even after a complete exhalation, there will still
be some residual air left in the lungs. There are equations
used to figure the probable residual air left in the lungs, and
these equations factor into the total equation so that residual
air does not appear to be body fat because of its buoyant
characteristics.

Underwater weighing is the most accurate method for determining body composition. It is currently the "gold standard" method for body weight as well as body composition
measurements. However, it is clearly not the most efficient
or widely available method for calculating body fat percent-

age. Not many people could afford the extremely expensive equipment or be able to fit it in their bathrooms. Even commercial gyms don't typically have underwater weighing tanks. To find one of these tanks, you would have to go to a university or medical research facility. Underwater weighing tanks are used almost exclusively for medical and nutrition research where a very high level of accuracy is required.

If you have any friends or family that claim to know their percentage of body fat, chances are that they were not assessed by underwater weighing, unless they participated in a research study. For the average person, body fat percentage can be measured at gyms or health fairs using a tool called a caliper.

In order to measure body fat by way of a caliper, a person needs both the tool as well as an individual trained to use the tool. It is not a measurement that you can take at home by yourself. Even a trained person cannot measure themselves accurately with a caliper; the process requires two people.

The technician who is doing the body fat measurements will "pinch" the fat on various parts of your body, like the stomach below the belly button, the backs of your arms, your calves, etc. The two sides of the caliper measure this pulled-out layer of adipose tissue. From each measurement, it is possible to estimate the body fat percentage for that part of the body. Most people have differing percentages in their legs, arms, and torso. Certain measurements can also be averaged together for an estimate of total body fat percentage.

When someone mentions their body fat percentage, this is probably what they are referring to. This figure is compared to the overall goals of 20% body fat for men and 30% body fat for women.

Body fat is an excellent tool for judging fitness over time as well. Many gyms and personal trainers make use of calipers to document and track their clients' body composition over time. Results are typically more consistent when the same technician performs the measurements. Each person tends to take the measurements in a slightly different way, which can lead to discrepancies. The best way to make use of calipers is to have the same individual check your body fat over time. For example, a trainer at your gym may check your body fat and tell you that your body is 42% fat. Afterward, you then work out for a couple of months at the gym. After this period of exercise, you go back to the same trainer, who at this point comes up with a measurement of 40% body fat. Because it was the same person performing the measurement both times, it is likely that you did, in fact, lose a couple of percentage points' worth of fat tissue. If, the week after your initial assessment, you had gone to a health fair in town and gotten someone else to measure your body fat and they told you were now at 40% body fat, it is more likely that this was due to the differing technicians and not your actual weight loss.

This is probably true because 1). you only worked out for a week, which is probably not long enough for your body to change very much, and 2). the body fat measurements done by different people do have a certain degree of variance. The caliper is no underwater weighing tank, but it is a good tool for the average person looking for a measure of their fitness level over time.

One of the main drawbacks of the caliper for measuring changes in the body is that it requires a trained person to assist you. You can't quickly take your own body fat measurements on a whim at two o'clock in the morning. Getting the measurement may require making an appointment at the gym or waiting for a health fair to be sponsored by the local hospital. It might cost you extra money to get this measurement done by a personal trainer. There is also a degree of invasion of privacy that many people don't like. Not only can you not do the measurement yourself, doing the measuring involves a stranger (or even worse- someone you know!) pinching your various fat reserves. Some people are willing to put up with it because they want the measurement. There are other people that you couldn't pay to submit themselves to this type of assessment. It is a personal decision whether a body fat assessment using a caliper is right for you. If it sounds uncomfortable, pick something else! There are plenty of options.

If you have zero access to an underwater weighing tank and aren't about to let anyone pinch anything, you can still get another type of assessment to determine your total body fat percentage. Another technique that has been developed for this very purpose is called bioelectrical impedance.

The scientific concept behind bioelectrical impedance is that various materials conduct electricity at various rates. Your first exposure to this concept was probably around age three, when your mother warned you not to stick metal utensils in the toaster because you could be electrocuted. Later on, you realized that you could stick wooden spoons in the toaster without harm because they didn't conduct electricity efficiently like metal does.

The body's tissues also conduct electricity at different rates. All in all, the human body clearly does conduct electricity, otherwise it wouldn't be possible for us to be electrocuted at all. There is, however, variance in the rates of conductivity between the lean and fatty tissues in the body. Fat impedes the flow of the electrical current more than the lean tissues do. The technique of bioelectrical impedance takes advantage of this fact. A weak electrical current is sent through the body. It's so weak that it isn't dangerous. The levels of impedance reveal what percentage of the body is composed of fat and what percentage is composed of lean tissue.

There are machines that measure the bioelectrical impedance. There are also scale-like implements on the popular market that send the electrical current through your feet when standing on the platform and then estimate your body fat percentage. The accuracy of such machines and scales depends largely on the brand and how much money was spent on the item. Bioelectrical impedance is a technique that can be used in research or medical situations, so there are machines that perform this method with a good level of accuracy.

One advantage to bioelectrical impedance is that it allows a bedridden individual to be weighed. If someone cannot stand on a scale or get into a tank of water or participate in percent fat estimation with a caliper, bioelectrical impedance can be a great option.

Between scales, articles of clothing, and various body-assessment machines, there are quite a few options for monitoring body weight over time. There are also other methods that could be individually developed for this purpose.

The important thing is not which method you pick, but that the method allows you to keep track of your progress over time. During the weight loss process, you need to know if your plan is working. If you are losing weight, or inches, or belt holes, or fat percentage, then you can be assured that you are on the right track. If you are not achieving the results that you want, it's time to go back to adjusting the personal calorie equation until the outcome turns around.

After you have successfully reached a comfortable weight, monitoring your weight is an important step to prevent the pounds from creeping back. Small increments of increase can serve as a warning that you are headed in the wrong direction and you will be able to adjust things before it becomes a more difficult problem.

So pick a way to monitor your weight. Maybe a combination

of a couple of methods would work best for you. Don't be obsessed with the numbers, but remember that if you have no objective measure, it will be hard to see change and easy to relapse!

CHAPTER 8

Simple Exercises that Help you Burn Calories Quickly

In previous chapters it has been established that although there are a handful of ways that the human body burns calories, the best way to increase calories burned is to increase daily physical activity. What constitutes "physical activity?" Basically, physical activity is any kind of body movement that you could possibly make. This includes everything from doing chores, cleaning your house, and walking your dog, to walking on a treadmill or climbing a mountain. All of these aforementioned activities, and any more activities that you can possibly come up with, burn calories. They don't burn calories at the same rates, but they all do burn more calories than doing nothing at all.

The hierarchy of calories burned per hour is an interesting
one. Sitting burns more calories than lying down. Sitting
and typing burns more calories than just sitting. Standing
burns more calories than sitting and typing. Walking burns
more calories than standing. This list of comparisons could
go on and on! Any movement will require your body to burn
calories for the energy to support the action. As a rule, the
more parts of your body that you move simultaneously, the
more calories you are going to burn per hour.

For example, imagine that you are typing furiously to complete a work assignment on time. The movement of your
fingers does burn calories, but your fingers don't really com-
prise a very large portion of your body. The total calories
burned are not that great. If you were to instead walk vig-
orously, this would be a much more effective method for
burning calories. Your legs are a much larger part of your
total body, so more calories are going to be required to fund
this movement. If you were swinging your arms while walking, you will do even better. If you were turning your head
or swinging your hips while you walked you would burn still
more calories. Of course, your terrible walking form may
cause an injury, so it probably isn't worth it. But the concept of more body motion causing more calorie usage is still
valid in this case.

Think of some activities that involve your entire body at one
time. Some great examples are walking, running, swimming,
biking, dancing, martial arts, and most team sports. These
are all fairly classic exercises because they engage the major-

ity of the body in action at one time. If you were to isolate a single motion from one of these activities, you would burn fewer calories. For example, if you were to sit in a chair and swing your arms as you would while walking, you wouldn't use nearly as many calories as walking, because your legs aren't involved. If you had poor balance or were unable to walk, then using your arms only for exercise might be a great option for you. You can still burn the same amount of calories, but it will take longer to do so.

Before you start into the business of picking and choosing activities that you enjoy and that burn the maximum amount of calories possible, there are some important issues for you to consider. If you have been inactive for a long period of time or are not sure about your fitness level, it is best to visit your primary care physician before you start any kind of new exercise routine. Your doctor will help you to define your personal limits to exercise safely. The goal is to get healthier, not injure yourself!

There are several tests that a physician can run to determine if there are potential concerns with your new plan for exercise. Checks include screenings for heart disease risk factors, like cholesterol and triglyceride levels and a blood pressure reading. A stress test is the most direct test of your physical fitness. Stress tests consist of supervised exercise during which a doctor monitors your various vital signs. In this way, he or she can judge how well your body reacts to various levels of strain and see if anything out of the ordinary is occurring.

Ask your doctor to help you to determine your target heart rate. Your target heart rate is the level of exertion at which you should attempt to exercise. Target heart rate depends on your age and physical condition. Heart rate is expressed in terms of beats per minute. If you know what your target heart rate should be, then you can find your pulse during exercise and count for one minute to see if you are near the target rate. If your count is higher than your target, you should probably cool it down a bit, and if your heart rate isn't high enough, you should try to work a little harder.

To burn the most possible calories in the least possible amount of time, you need to make your body work as hard as it can within its own limits. (And to reiterate : working past your physical limits is a bad idea because it can cause bad things to happen. "Bad things" would be events like muscle strains, heart attacks, passing out, or just feeling like crap.)

One factor already mentioned is the percentage of the total body that is engaged in the activity. If more of your body is working, more calories will be burned. The next factor to consider is your level of exertion during the activity. Strolling slowly burns less calories than a brisk walk. Treading water just to keep yourself afloat is going to use less calories than if you tread water furiously enough to keep your shoulders out of the water. This factor follows common sense. Work harder at any given activity and you will burn more calories.

Finding the balance between being comfortable and using

as many calories as possible can be difficult. Consider two activities: walking down the street at your normal pace, and sprinting up the side of a mountain while carrying a ninety pound bag of sand. You don't have to be a genius to figure out which one of these options burns more calories per hour. However, which one would you choose to do? How many more days per week are you likely to complete the walk than the sprint? This is where it all gets tricky. If you do the sprint one time this year, but would walk four times a week all year, you would actually end up burning many more calories walking than you would sprinting.

Please heavily factor in your commitment to any given activity. If you won't do it regularly, it doesn't really matter how many calories you theoretically could burn if you did. Some people would rather run for fifteen minutes than walk for an hour. To these people, time is the most important factor in their exercise. They would rather do it and be done. Although it depends on their walking and running speeds, it is reasonable to assume that an hour of walking and fifteen minutes of running could take the same amount of total calories.

There are plenty of other people who would take the long walk hands down. Maybe they find walking relaxing, or maybe they just hate running and are willing to invest the time to avoid it altogether. It doesn't matter which camp you fall into, but be honest with yourself so that you don't make an exercise program that you hate.

Exercise at the highest level of exertion that is safe for you and that you can personally deal with on a long-term basis. If you can speed up your walking a little bit, then do it! More calories are used when you walk at the faster pace. Most people are surprised that walking is a great exercise that can help you lose weight. Somehow, it doesn't seem like "hard enough" exercise to do anything. Sure, swimming the butterfly will burn more calories per minute, but with walking you typically reap the advantages of consistency. Is a professional swimmer going to be in better shape than someone who walks thirty minutes a day? Of course, but someone walking a half hour each day is in much better shape than someone who isn't. The trick is consistency. If you walk for thirty minutes a day, you will be continuously putting those minuses into your calorie equation.

Thirty minutes is actually an excellent activity goal to shoot for. The Surgeon General currently recommends that everyone does something physically active for thirty minutes on most days of the week. This level will help you to be generally physically fit. If you are trying to lose weight, the recommendations increase to sixty to ninety minutes of activity five times a week. This might sound like a lot, but considering that you need to burn five hundred calories a day to lose one pound a week, it makes perfect sense. Remember that you don't need to start out at that level of activity. It can be something to work up to. And again, doing something, anything, more than what you are currently doing is going to be an improvement.

All of the Surgeon General's recommendations are for total exercise throughout the day. You could ride your bike for fifteen minutes to work and back and take a thirty-minute walk on your lunch break and that would count as sixty minutes. For many people, smaller chunks of activity fit better into their schedules than one hour-long or hour-and-a-half-long session . That's okay; it's up to you to decide how you can best fit your activity into your lifestyle.

The Surgeon General's recommendations are something for you to try to work up to in the future, not something that you have to start with this afternoon. If you begin with an exercise routine that is longer than your current physical capabilities, then you won't keep up with it consistently. And as it has been mentioned a few times before, consistency over the long-term is the trick to losing weight.

There are a couple of good ways to make sure that you will be consistent with your activity. First, choose an activity that is not overly challenging for you. If you associate your workout with pain, then you aren't going to do it regularly. You will probably spend more time thinking of excuses to get out of your activity than you will actually exercising! That's a bad sign.

Next, be sure to pick an appropriate length of time to do the activity. Maybe walking is a reasonable activity for you. Four-hour long walks are most likely too far though. The level of activity is right for you, but you've chosen a poor length. This can also work in the opposite way. If you are a reasonably fit person, there is no reason to start your walking routine at a length of 2 minutes! If you can walk for 20 minutes or a half an hour, then do that.

Finally, to maximize your consistency, pick an activity that you enjoy. There are some things in life that you will never have time to do. No matter how bored you are, there is always something that sounds better than it. Maybe it bores you, aggravates you, disinterests you, or frustrates you. Whatever the reason, you will probably be eternally "too busy" to get to whatever it is. Now if that activity is the kind of exercise you plan on doing, you are setting yourself up for failure.

Sometimes it's hard to tell which activities you actually like and which activities you just wish that you liked. A good way to determine that for yourself is this: if someone asked you to do the activity right now, would you want to? If you would, great. If you instead answered something more along the lines of "well, I just, you know, need to do some stuff.... But this weekend might work out better," then you had better pick something else for your activity. Come this weekend, something else will come up and you still won't get out and do your exercise.

Exercising regularly can be challenging enough without try-ing to make yourself do something that you dislike. Pick something that you enjoy and want to make time for in your life. Be creative: is there anything that you would be in the mood for regularly? If you like to dance, turn on your music or the radio every day and dance for a certain amount of minutes. There's no reason that dancing should only be relegated to wedding receptions. If you like to people-watch or get out of the house, then take your walks at the mall. If there is some type of class at the gym that you could get excited about, sign up for it. If you need to make a bet about your fitness with yourself, or your brother, or your friend to be motivated, then do it.

Once you have determined with the help of your doctor a level of exercise that is safe for you, picked a general activity (hopefully one that requires full-body movement, so that you can burn the most calories), and picked a length of time that is reasonable for you to do this activity, you are almost ready to go. In fact, you could go out and get started right now, but there are still a couple more words of advice to help you use up the most calories possible during your workout. To maximize the calorie-burning potential of any activity there is a little trick that can be thrown in during the workout. This fitness technique is popularly known as "interval training." It sounds very high-tech, but the concept is simple. In this workout method, you will do several alternating intervals of easier and harder exercise.

To understand this idea, let's look at the classic example of a runner running around a track. Maybe the runner's normal pace is about a nine-minute mile. If the runner were just going to go on a simple run without using intervals, he or she might run three miles in about twenty seven minutes. His or her pace wouldn't vary during the entirety of the workout.

However, if the runner wanted to do intervals, he or she would start out at the typical pace, run a lap, then run faster for a lap, then go back to normal pace for another lap, then pick up the pace again, etc. The intervals wouldn't necessarily have to be a lap long. The runner might run two laps at regular pace, then run faster for thirty seconds, or one hundred meters, or fifty meters, or from one landmark to another. As the person working out, the runner is in charge of determining how long and how many intervals there are going to be.

There are many advantages to intervals. First of all, they make your workout a bit more interesting. There is nothing like doing a repetitive action for a half hour to bore you or put you to sleep (and you can't sleep, because you are running!)

Another nice thing about intervals is that your body gets to practice working harder, but it doesn't have to stay there for a long time. Say our runner usually gets to a speed of seven and a half minute miles during intervals. This is much more work than going nine minute miles. The runner probably is not capable of doing seven and a half minute miles for a long time period. However, running at that higher speed gets the runner's body into better shape than just going at the comfortable nine-minute mile pace. By pushing during those short periods, your body starts to get to the next level of fitness, rather than getting into a rut.

The next really nice thing about intervals is that they are

fairly comfortable. The rhythm of your workout is "rest, push, rest, push, rest." Unlike a workout that is just flat-out hard to do, you get some time at a comfortable pace to catch your breath after you've finished an interval.

And finally, intervals help to burn more calories than working out at a steady pace. By increasing your effort during the interval periods, you burn calories at a higher rate. Also, many exercisers find that they can go longer when they do intervals. This translates into more calories used. Maybe you can't really run very far, so you choose to walk. If you were to walk for a mile, that would be good exercise. If you continue to walk a mile every day, but start doing three intervals of twenty seconds of jogging during the walk, it is even better exercise. You will burn more calories, and you are training your body to be able to work harder so that you could eventually switch to running if you wanted to.

The beauty of intervals is that they apply to any activity that you can do for exercise. The concept is easy to explain in the context of running, but intervals aren't just for runners. If you are walking, you can walk faster during your intervals. If you are dancing, you can dance harder during your intervals. If you are using any machine at the gym, you can go up a couple of levels of difficulty during your intervals. If you are on a treadmill, you can increase the incline for your intervals. If you play soccer or basketball, rush the other team or sprint across the field/court for an interval. Whatever your preferred activity, you can add intervals to burn more calories.

You now have your very own outline for burning the most possible calories. Pick an activity that is safe for you; do this activity for the longest time period and at the highest exertion that is safe and reasonable for you. Add intervals to kick your workout up a notch. And be consistent with this program over time so that you can reap the weight-loss results of all of your activity.

CHAPTER 9

How to Exercise in your Daily Life

A lot of people are afraid of the word "exercise." For some, it conjures up bad images of the 1980s, bodysuits, and step aerobics. It is uncomfortable for these people to even think about participation in so-called exercise.

Luckily, exercise has moved out of the realm of big socks and bad exercise videos. Even more luckily is that you don't even really, truly need to exercise to be fit or to lose weight.

What? How could anyone possibly say such a thing?

The most lucky thing of all is that exercise specialists now recognize the value of something referred to as "physical activity." Physical activity is any possible motion that your body can do. At first glance, this might seem suspiciously close to exercise, but consider the vast differences. Exercise is an intentional motion to train and condition the body. You exercise in a gym; running laps and doing push-ups and crunches is exercise. During exercise, you are essentially running on a human version of a gerbil wheel. With exercise you aren't going anywhere. You are working an awful lot, but you aren't doing anything. The end result is that your body has used calories. It will burn fat and build more muscle and you will be more fit. For the purpose that it is intended, exercise is just great. It does exactly what it promises.

However, what about all of those activities that actually are productive? What about when you push a heavy grocery cart around the store? What about raking your leaves or pushing a kid on a swing? How about picking up things around your house or walking to your boss's office? These activities and literally countless others are not undertaken with the same intention as exercise. You are doing them to complete a task- you want food for the house or you need to discuss a project with your supervisor. Because you had not exclusively intended to condition your body when you began these activities, they don't count as exercise. Motions that are not exercise are instead classified as physical activity. However, the interesting thing is that the physical outcome is fairly similar. Calories are burned, the body is conditioned, and the body becomes more fit.

There was a time when humans didn't even have exercise. It was something that was invented somewhere along the line. Before there was exercise, there was only physical activity.

Physical activity alone was responsible for the physical fitness of the population. And physical activity did just fine. Our bodies can't really tell if we are doing a productive action or just exercise. The body is just going to fund your motion with energy from calories, and then its job is complete. Maybe you are running on a treadmill facing a big mirrored wall at your local gym. Maybe you are running after a bison trying to stab it with a spear so that you can eat it. To your body, it's pretty much the same deal.

In fact, exercise had to be invented at some point to mimic all of the activities that humans had stopped having to do. Driving replaced walking and fast food drive-thrus replaced hunting and gathering. No wonder we found ourselves falling a little behind in our calorie usage. Everyday life just isn't quite as physically challenging as it used to be.

Physical activity can vary considerable between individuals, especially with respect to their profession. People who work labor-intensive jobs get a lot more physical activity each day than people who work in offices on computers. Walking, lifting, reaching, and walking around some more really burns a lot of calories throughout the day. Even standing versus sitting can make a fair difference, as in the case of a classroom teacher compared with a school administrator. Jobs make a big difference in daily physical activity.

Having an active job doesn't guarantee fitness and health. It's still possible to gain weight f you are eating more calories than you are expending. Active people can always benefit from exercise or additional physical activity as well.

If you have a sedentary job, it is even more important for you to take time each day to exercise or to significantly increase your physical activity level. A sedentary lifestyle puts you at a huge disadvantage as far as losing or maintaining body weight. Non-activity means that your overall calorie requirements are not very high. Plan to increase your calories burned, whether by exercise or physical activity.

Increasing your daily physical activity is kind of like a game. It's a game with fairly high stakes because you are playing for a longer life expectancy, lower risk of disease, looking sexy in your pants, etc. You want to be doing good at this game! One thing worth nothing about this game, though, is that it requires reversing your thinking on a little topic called efficiency.

You have probably been playing the efficiency game with yourself since childhood. Efficiency entails always finding the easiest and faster and least painful method for accomplishing any task. It might require setting up a system or protocol of some kind, or even building a new machine to help with the task. Sometimes efficiency just requires some ingenuity in determining task order. If you have ever done anything such as grabbing a trashcan at the bottom of the driveway while you go by on the riding mower so that you can avoid an extra trip, you know exactly what I'm talking about. Think of all of the contraptions and schemes that you've come up with over the years in order to reduce your physical

workload. Some people are even paid to figure this type
of thing out for major corporations: they are employed as
efficiency engineers.

If you make your living by planning efficient processes, it is
probably best to continue to think that way at work. However, to increase your level of daily physical activity, you
will have to do the exact opposite in every personal situation. Undoing your very makeup may feel strange at first,
but you'll get used to it quickly, especially since you know
that it is for such a good cause. Plus, the non-efficiency game
can be every bit as addicting as the efficiency game. Soon
you will be doing everything you do in the worst possible
way, all in the name of your waistline.

In this whole new paradigm of non-efficiency, some things
will have to go. Machines are first on the list. If it is a labor-
saving device, try to avoid using it as much as possible. You
have taken that machine into your home out of the kindness
of your heart and it only returns the favor by cheating you
out of burned calories. It's incredible.

Not only should you downgrade your riding mower to a push-
mower (or even better, a pair of scissors), you should be
carrying the trashcans to the house one at a time so that
you will be getting in a few more steps. That's right. Even
if you are burly enough to hoist all five over your shoulder at
the same time, take the long route and do one single trashcan
at a time.

If you think about it, situations like this are a gold mine of inefficiency. Think about carrying the groceries into the house from the trunk of the car. Efficiency says to park as close to the house as possible and then try to grab all of the bags at once for a single trip. What if you parked farther away and carried the bags in one by one? Your neighbors might think you were a little crazy, if they even notice your grocery-carrying habits. (It might be a little vain to suppose that they would.) Otherwise, nothing changes except it takes you two minutes longer to unload the groceries, and you burn several more calories in the process. It doesn't really make you that much later. It doesn't really make you that much more tired. All in all, it is probably a reasonably good deal. It's a good deal that you should be taking advantage of whenever possible.

Take the non-efficiency idea further. Try to let it permeate every area of your life. Let no action go unscrutinized. Analyze every action that you do tomorrow, and then think of several ways that you could make that action less physically efficient. Then try to think of ways to push it even further. Try not to think of this as a waste of your time, but as making small payments on your daily exercise instead of paying in one lump sum. Remind yourself continuously that by doing everything the least efficient way possible, you are getting out of having to do concentrated chunks of traditional exercise. And, after all, you need to somehow non-efficiency your way into using up enough calories to approximate the energy used during one buffalo hunt and several hours of tool-less farming, because that's what your daily physical activity may have consisted of a couple thousand years ago. Remember that.

Rethinking your current systems for completing activities is one thing, but increasing the amount of steps that you take each day is another interesting subdivision of the whole concept of increasing your activity through non-efficiency.

Whole books could be written about increasing daily steps. It might even be an easier game than the non-efficiency game, because it has one basic strategy: take the longest route possible between where you started at and where you are trying to get to. The step-increasing people do things like always taking the stairs and parking in the farthest parking spots available it their company's parking lots so that they have to walk longer to get to their cubicles. An active step-increaser would figure out where the farthest bathroom in the building is, and then make a point to use it regularly. A real pro might only fill his or her water bottle up halfway at the water cooler, so as to make more trips to the cooler to get refills, and the beauty of a good water intake is that you have even more opportunity to make use of the far-away bathroom!

Communications are also an excellent time to get more steps in. Sure you could call or email someone in the office, but that isn't a very good calorie rate per hour. Walking over to deliver messages personally (and then taking the long way back to your desk) is much more effective, calorie-wise.

Luckily, there are tools available to assist someone who is attempting to increase his or her daily steps. Pedometers are devices that count each step taken while the pedometer is worn. Some models even calculate total distance covered by judging your stride length and then multiplying by the total amount of steps that were taken.

Some people use pedometers while they are out exercising, say, out on a walk. This is helpful because the pedometer tells you how much ground you've covered. It's kind of like another sports watch in some ways. Pedometers probably aren't being used to their full potential if they are just used for measuring walks. Physical activity is so much tougher to quantify because it is very spread out throughout the day, so a pedometer can probably give you even more information if you are using it for this purpose.

To judge your total daily activity using a pedometer, you need to be wearing it for the majority of your day. Try to remember to put it on when you first put your clothes on in the morning. If you tend to do some things around the house in your pajamas before you get dressed, then this is not a good time for you. Try to put it on as quickly as possible so that you don't miss any steps that you take.

Most pedometers either go in your pocket or clip onto your waistband like pager holders or cell phone holders. From the swinging motion of your leg throughout the day, the pedometer estimates your total steps taken. Some pedometers are more accurate than others. There are many moderately priced pedometers that are accurate. If you have doubts about yours, you can test it by walking a known distance or counting a certain number of steps and then comparing it to your pedometer's estimate. There are also websites devoted to comparisons of various pedometers, so you can look up an accurate brand and model before you purchase one.

There are also guidelines for physical activity as measured by pedometers to assist you. The Surgeon General has recognized the validity of physical activity in place of exercise, and recommends that everyone try for at least 10,000 steps per day. He has said that this is approximately equivalent to a half hour of exercise. So each person can choose between a half hour of exercise on four or more days of the week and walking 10,000 steps throughout the day most days of the week. That might sound like a complete deal, but keep in mind that the average American only walks about half of that figure. Over the whole country, 5,000 steps is more or less the norm. And of course, there are plenty of people who fall very much below this average who are counterbalanced by some super-active people on the other end.

If you decide that counting steps would help to motivate you to be more active on a daily basis, then a good idea is to first figure out what your personal baseline is. Your baseline in this case just means the amount of steps that you typically take in a day. It's a good idea to know where you are starting from before you attempt improvement. Wear your pedometer all day every day for one week and record the amount of steps that you end up with each day. Don't try to increase at this point; you are just trying to figure out what you are starting out with.

The next step is to Take the week's worth of daily step totals and add them together and divide this number by seven. You now have the weekly average. How did it turn out? Did you get over the national average? Under the national average? Are you close to the 10,000 steps?

Wherever your baseline ends up, don't be discouraged. Just focus on increasing your daily steps by small increments. For example, if your baseline was 2,000 steps per day, try to get at least 2,500 steps every day the next week. The week after that, shoot for 3,000. Work your way up until you get at least 10,000 steps with regularity. Notice which days you tend to get the most steps and which days you tend to get the least steps. Are your high-step days when you go shopping, or when you do projects around the house? When you have a long meeting, does that tend to take a chunk out of your steps? Are you much more sedentary on the weekends than on the weekdays? Use this information to help you to increase your steps on the hard days. If you have a meeting scheduled, then realize that you will probably have to take a walk later in the day to make up for the step loss. If you get stumped on ways to get more steps, see http://www.smallstep.gov/ for more lists of suggestions that you can use.

Increasing your steps can also be combined with inefficient tasking and regular exercise to maximize your calorie burning capacity. It was previously discussed that many people need sixty to ninety minutes of exercise most days of the week. Remember that 10,000 steps counts as one half hour of exercise. If you continually reach the 10,000 step goal and then do another thirty minutes of activity or of exercise, you can easily reach the hour mark.

Planning for inefficiency and using a pedometer can help you to increase your daily physical activity. That's the point. However, try not to lose sight of your overall goal. The only reason you are making use of these tools is to use up more calories each day to help with your weight loss or weight maintenance. It doesn't really matter if you have a pedometer or not; the important thing is that you are taking the steps!

CHAPTER 10

Eating Good Food, with Less Calories

Knowing that you need to reduce your calorie intake and actually achieving that reduction are two very different things. There are many obstacles that can come up during the quest to cut calories over time. One main concern that many dieters have is whether or not they will be able to continue eating "good" food as they lose weight. While "good" is certainly a very subjunctive word, chances are that you will continue to enjoy eating the foods that you enjoy while you are in the weight loss process, as well as once you reach the point of weight maintenance. There is no reason that you would need to spontaneously adopt a diet that consists of only celery, air, and rice cakes just because you want to lose weight.

In fact, assuring that your lower-calorie food tastes great

is very important. Just as you are unlikely to maintain an exercise routine that you hate, you are equally as unlikely to consistently eat foods that you dislike. Consistency is vital to your weight loss effort. The personal calorie equation has to go in your favor every day to successfully lose pounds. Use good food as your ally, not your torturer!

When planning ways to eat good foods that have less calories, one of the most important things to do first is to analyze what it exactly is that you currently eat. Changing your habits is hard if you have absolutely no idea what those habits are. Your analysis may as informal as just keeping the idea in the back of your mind over the next couple of days and paying attention to what you put in your mouth throughout the day. Your analysis could also be a bit more formal.

A formal analysis would require you to write down everything that you eat for a day or two, or even up to week. All beverages, snacks, desserts, "tastes," and meals should be recorded. If you chew a piece of gum, put it on the list. If you have a cough drop, put that down. That might sound a bit overboard, but if you are going to do a formal analysis of your eating habits, you may as well do it the right way. Plus, you may actually gain a fair amount of your calories from tasting other peoples' food or grabbing a bite here and a couple of crackers there. If you don't include everything, you'll never know.

Once you have a written list of what you ate and drank and

nibbled on for the chosen time period, give your list a quick, informal once-over to try to gain some basic insight. You may notice things such as your tendency to skip breakfast and lunch altogether. Maybe you will notice that you didn't eat a vegetable in three days. Maybe you will be surprised at the percentage of your meals and snacks that consist of breakfast cereal. (That's not necessarily a bad thing, just an observation.)

Now it's time for the real analysis. Use a nutrition program to calculate your calorie and vitamin and mineral intake. There are several of these types of programs available on the web, such as the "My Pyramid Tracker" program, which can be found at `http://www.mypyramid.gov`. This analysis will show you the amount of calories that you ate during the recorded period, and also suggest food groups that you should eat more or less of in order to achieve a balanced diet. It can be really helpful information.

Your analysis, whether formal or informal, will give you some helpful clues on how to go about changing your diet for the better. One really important consideration is which foods you cannot live without. Think back or look back through your list for the last few days. What are the highest-calorie foods that you eat regularly? Are there certain routines that you have concerning food, such as going out to eat at a certain restaurant with friends once a week? Maybe you tend to eat a certain food every day for a snack, or for breakfast. You probably also have traditional family foods that you like to make, especially on holidays.

These are all important foods because they are things that probably will always be in your life. That's a good thing; food is cultural and food is entertainment. When you start making changes in your eating you wouldn't want to have to change your culture and your entertainment at the same time! That is probably an uphill battle that you're not going to win.

There are also probably lots of other high-calorie foods that are merely part of your diet for convenience reasons. These are the things that you grab because someone else makes them available to you or because you don't have time to wait for a lower-calorie option. Consider this type of high-calorie foods in another category.

So by now you should have all of the high-calorie foods that you eat regularly separated into two categories. There is a "I love it, can't live with out it " category, and the "well, it's just there" category. They are all comprised of high-calorie foods, but they will get treated very differently in your low-calorie eating plan.

The "love it" category includes your all-time favorite foods, family foods, and comfort foods. Maybe you love bacon. Maybe a bowl of ice cream is your favorite thing. Maybe it's a cold regular soda or fried rice from the Chinese restaurant down the street. It could be pepperoni pizza that just hits the spot. Whatever that food is that you love, you need to be sure to include it in your diet regularly. The main reasons for this are 1.) to make you happy, and 2.) to keep you from going crazy and binging on large quantities of this food after you've tried to avoid it for awhile. If you try to give up your favorite foods altogether, you won't be successful.

You are not going to give up any of your favorite foods, because that is a ridiculous proposition, but because they are high-calorie, you can't exactly eat them all day every day either. Ultimately it all comes down to moderation and portion size. There is no reason to swear off all "bad foods." There is a saying that goes, "There are no bad foods, only bad quantities." This could be the theme of your "love it" category. You are going to continue to eat those high-calorie foods that you love, but limit them so they don't prevent your weight loss.

Decide on a reasonable amount of this food to eat. Maybe you like bacon every morning. That daily habit takes a big chunk of your daily calories, plus all of the saturated fat is pretty hard on your heart and arteries. How about eating just one or two strips one morning on the weekend? That's true moderation. This type of restraint can be applied to any high-calorie foods that you like, from cheese puffs to grandma's fudge.

The high-calorie foods that ended up in your "don't care" list will be treated very differently than the foods in your "love it" list. Most people spend a lot of their daily calories on foods that don't particularly bring them much pleasure. It's a shame. It's a waste. These calories are heavy in the calorie equation, and they don't really make you very happy when you eat them. Make a conscious effort not to eat things just because they are present. This is more a habit than anything. However, it is a habit that makes it hard for you to lose weight.

Try to think of some examples in your own life where you tend to eat calories that aren't really worth it. If you eat the stale, broken, day-old donut pieces out of the box in the employee break room just because they are there, this is exactly what I'm talking about! If donuts are on the "love" list, you can have them. But eat ONE, and make it a good one since it is your only one. Make it one that's fresh from the bakery and is your very favorite flavor. Those old stale ones are a waste because they don't give you the maximum enjoyment on your calorie investment. Can you believe that stale donuts have the same amount of calories as fresh donuts? It almost doesn't seem fair, does it?

On the other hand, let's say that you tend to eat the stale donuts at work, but donuts aren't even on your personal "love" list. This situation could be even more tragic. If you really don't care about donuts, then don't eat them. Save your calories for a cold beer, or some homemade cookies, or macaroni and cheese from the box, or a round of late-night nachos and a burrito, or a piece of chocolate cake, or whatever it is that you like best. It only makes sense.

The next change that you might want to consider in order to reduce calories but still enjoy your food is to change the proportions eaten of different foods throughout your day.

Say you typically fill your dinner plate half-full with a meat entrée, then add several spoons of potatoes (with cheese and butter on them), and then put two lonely green beans on the side of your plate in the last available location. To change the proportions, you need to stop eating five or six times larger quantities of high-calorie foods than the low-calorie foods that you eat. In this dinner situation, the green beans are the lower-calorie item, and the meat and potatoes are a toss-up.

Switch everything around on the dinner plate. You don't even have to cook a different dinner to do this trick! Just start with the vegetable (which is almost guaranteed to be the lowest-calorie item on the table, unless it is drenched in butter or cream sauce or cheese). Fill your plate half-full or one-third full of green beans, and there will be a little less room for meat and potatoes. Meat and potatoes are fine, just in smaller portions. If you always begin your meals by filling your plate half full with fruits and/or vegetables or other low-calorie foods, your overall calories eaten will probably be less than they are currently. It will be less calories, but still be the food that you know and love.

Another tip is to be sure to avoid the "stupid" high-calorie foods. These are similar to the high-calorie foods that you don't like in that they just aren't worth eating. The difference between the "stupid" high-calorie foods and the high-calorie foods that you don't care for is that "stupid" high-calorie foods masquerade as harmless, low-calorie foods. The stupid foods are the ones that aren't really even that exciting, but tend to have a lot of fat or sugar or something that makes them high in calories. These foods are very sneaky.

These are the foods that no one realizes are so high-calorie. You have to be somewhat vigilant and check food labels every once in a while to make sure that you aren't eating one of these stupid foods. An example of one common stupid food is the fattening, extremely high-calorie crackers available out there. Yes, crackers. They are the same crackers that you plan to crunch up and put in your soup where they will turn to mush. It's pretty pointless to spend your calories there. And if you aren't paying attention to it, you could use several hundred calories in one handful of crackers. Look instead for some fat-free crackers. The weird thing is that, in soup, it honestly all tastes the same. Read the food labels of things that you normally buy to screen for these types of tricksters.

You've already figured out which high-calorie foods you can't live without, and which high-calorie foods you should just toss, but what about the rest of the lower-calorie food that you are eating each day? What are the most delicious ways to go about lighter eating ?

Flavor is a good place to start. A common complaint about low-calorie foods is their blandness. Low-calorie foods aren't inherently bland. However, if your only techniques for adding flavor to foods are frying the food, adding oil, adding butter, or adding cheese... well, no wonder you aren't making any flavorful low-calorie foods!

There are lots of flavor-enhancing agents besides added fats. If you aren't aware of any of these, don't be too hard on yourself. A lot of traditional "American" food that originated in Europe relies solely on fat and salt to make it taste good. It may be that you just honestly haven't had many foods flavored in any other way. That's okay; now is a really good time to start. Go to your spice cabinet. Look inside. Take note of all of the spices that you have available to cook with or to put on food that has already been prepared. If you could not complete this request either because you do not have a spice cabinet/drawer/shelf, or because that cabinet/drawer/shelf only contains salt and pepper, then you may have to do a bit of background research first.

Here are some recommendations to help you discover the joy of spices. First, go to an Italian restaurant. Don't order anything with alfredo sauce, because that it just butter and salt and won't help you to grow at all during this exercise. Order something with marinara sauce (tomato sauce) and order a salad with Italian dressing. While you eat, think about what the food tastes like. The sauce doesn't taste like a plain tomato, does it? And the salad doesn't taste like a plain piece of lettuce, does it? There are a lot of different spices at work in these two dishes to cause you to taste their particular flavors. Common spices used in Italian cuisine are oregano, basil, parsley, and garlic. Salads are often made with balsamic vinegar and spices. To recreate these flavors, you will need to have these spices, or at least an Italian spice mix, available in your kitchen.

The next stop (on a different day, of course; you wouldn't want to go over your calorie needs for the day) is going to be a Mexican restaurant. A small mom-and-pop place is going to be better than a commercial chain. The chains often cater to the cheese, oil, and salt crowd, so you won't learn anything about spices there. If you can find a more authentic Mexican restaurant, chances are that there will be grilled foods, spicy foods, and lots of lime juice. In Mexico it is common to use lime juice to flavor corn on the cob, salad, popcorn, beans, peanuts, and tequila.. Try lime juice on something you like to eat. It is good for you and definitely adds a new flavor. Some Tabasco or chili powder is quite noticeable as well.

Finally, make sure you visit a good Indian restaurant. Indian cuisine may be the king of spice combining. Besides curry, there are usually so many different spices in the different dishes that it is hard to identify any one individual spice. It might be best to find some Indian recipes if you want to recreate this flavor!

Italian, Mexican, and Indian cuisine are three types of spice-loving cuisines that are commonly found in the United States. There are many, many more. Look around your house. When someone cooks a new dish for you that you like, be sure to ask what spices they used to prepare it. If you find it intimidating to use individual spices, buy pre-made spice mixes. They are a bit more foul-proof. If you can find spice mixes without salt added, those are best. Then you can add as much spice as you like without making the food too salty. You can add salt separately anyway. Be sure to try things like microwaving frozen vegetables and then adding spices to them. That makes a very flavorful, low-calorie side dish. Your vegetables will go from wet and mushy to pretty delicious.

The perfect companion to your new stock of spices is a set of non-stick cooking pans. Non-stick pans have the advantage of not needing butter or oil or anything in the bottom when you cook with them. That oil that you put in the bottom of the pan to keep everything from sticking doesn't make the food taste that much better, but it does add calories. Saving a couple of teaspoons or tablespoons of fat every time that you cook something can add up over time.

You now have the tools to make good-tasting and low-calorie food for yourself. This whole thing probably isn't going to be as bad as you thought it might be. Eat the high-calorie foods that you love, but do so in moderation. Base your diet on the lowest-calorie of all foods: fruits and vegetables. When you cook, add flavor to foods with a variety of spices instead of just using oil, butter, cheese, and salt. Cook these foods in non-stick pans to avoid having to use fat during the cooking process. With a little practice, your light food will be delicious!

CHAPTER 11

Keeping Up when Things Get Tough

If you have recently set out on your weight loss journey, talking about the tough times is probably something that you don't want to do right now. You feel good. You feel motivated. Your plan is surely foul proof. In fact, you might think that this isn't so hard at all.

This is a great attitude, however, it is important to be realistic and to know that anytime you set out to do something long-term, there are going to be some tough times. For human beings, the only possible way to avoid problems at any given activity or interaction is to shorten the length of the activity so that it is over before any conflict can occur. Of course, this strategy only works on a very selected range of activities. Most likely you have already pushed this strategy to the limits in other areas of your life.

The thing about weight loss is that it is going to be a life-long change. First you change your habits in order to lose the weight, and then you keep up those habits and adjust as necessary to maintain your weight throughout the rest of your life. It's a great goal. It is definitely achievable, but knowing that tough times will come is important. Then once they do come (it's inevitable), you won't feel like you have failed. A few obstacles, setbacks, and moves in the wrong direction do not mean failure. They are just the challenges that go along with any worthy long-term goal.

Luckily, since you have been forewarned about the coming of these setbacks, you have an advantage. You have a head start on the problems that will try to catch up with you during the whole weight-loss process. If you strategize now, you will be all the more prepared for whatever comes your way during your weight loss battle.

One thing that is fairly predictable about obstacles is that they repeat themselves. One person isn't hit with a variety of obstacles, but typically faces essentially the same issue over and over and over again. It can be quite maddening, actually. However, the repetitive nature of your obstacles allows you to predict them before they actually occur. It's pretty tricky, actually.

Think of any past times when you may have tried to lose weight. Here you are right now, trying to lose it again, so something must have turned out differently that you planned the first time. What was the obstacle that kept you from reaching your goal? Did you give up and stop caring? Maybe you got really busy at work and then it got pushed to the back burner. Maybe you lost weight, but then it crept back up again. Maybe your last weight loss plan wasn't implemented long enough for you to actually see any results. Maybe you tend to eat when you are stressed, and you had a very stressful year that year. The reasons vary from person to person, but you should know your own obstacles better than anybody. It can be frustrating to think about this, but remember that you are only doing this now to avoid being ambushed again by your previous attackers. Seriously, they have done this to you before.

More clues can be gleaned from other things that you have struggled with during your life. Don't cast your analysis solely on weight loss attempts. Think of other hard things that you've done. Did you quit smoking? Are you married? Did you rebuild a car or build a computer from parts? Did you start a new career? What kinds o f problems did you come across during these endeavors? The activity doesn't so much matter; you are just trying to identify typical obstacles for yourself.

Once you have come up with the main ways that you usually get distracted, discouraged, or bored, you have a definite start. You are on the right track to heading off your obstacles before they even appear. Try to think about ways that these past obstacles could come up again in your current life.

There are some of these obstacles that are recurring as well.

From where you are right now, what can you see that could be a future challenge? It could be far off in the future, or it could be next week. Do you think that it will be hard to be active during the wintertime? Do you tend to live exclusively on large chunks of fatty meats and beer during grilling-out season? Does one of your roommates or your partner do the grocery shopping and tend to do a very high-calorie job of it? Do you dine with people who shun vegetables? If these are problems for you, you probably already know it, or at least you are thinking about it now that it's been brought up.

You probably have a realistic idea of the obstacles that you will face as you try to be more active, eat healthier, and lose weight. You are the only person truly qualified to address these obstacles. Only you know what the obstacles are like, and what solutions you can truly live with. Start with a plan for each of your foreseen obstacles. What kinds of things could you do during the winter for activity? Could you go to the store with the family grocery shopper, or at least put some requests on the list? What will you do during grilling season anyway? These are all worth pondering.

Inevitably, of course, many more obstacles will come your way that were not foreseen. That's why it is a very good thing that you have already been practicing how to overcome obstacles to achieve your health plans. Suppose you u have been happily and successfully losing weight. You've been eating right and going to a group fitness training class a the local gym. Overall, you feel pretty good. Then one week,

you start to feel sort of sluggish. You miss one class and start
to drag every time you think about getting ready to go to the
gym for the class. At this point, a common reaction might
be to give up, quit, and say that it probably wasn't possible
for you to lose weight anyway. Some people also tend to
berate themselves for not doing a better job of keeping up
with it.

All of these approaches are pointless. You will lose the effort
you have already invested in the project, you won't continue
to lose weight as you had planned, and you may start to feel
worse about yourself. Those are all good reasons to approach
obstacles from a different angle. When you notice the very
first signs of hesitation about your physical activity or your
nutrition choices, stop and think about the situation.

First, identify the real obstacle that you are facing. Why
don't you want to go to the class any more? Be honest with
yourself. Maybe it is too hard. Maybe it is too easy. Maybe
you don't like the instructor. Maybe driving over there to
the gym takes too long and then you don't get to see your
family as much as you'd like. Maybe you are just bored
because you have been doing the same class for a long time.
Notice how the problem looks much more solvable when it
is broken down. Your overall reaction might have originally
been to scrap the whole thing, but the solution is easier than
that. Maybe you need to switch classes or just do a different
kind of physical activity altogether. Whatever the solution,
it is not nearly as drastic as quitting your fitness goals in
their entirety. Frustration will come, but try to think of

solutions that go right to the root of the true problem.

For many people who have lost weight or are currently losing weight, there is one stage that is dreaded. It is commonly referred to as a "weight-loss plateau." All that really means is that you are stuck. Your weight is no longer going up or down, but has flat-lined. You've already lost weight, and you want to lose more, but it doesn't seem to be happening. Your old tricks don't seem to work any more. You are doing the exact same thing that you used to do, except back then you were losing a pound a week.

It can be an incredibly frustrating time for someone who is working hard to lose weight. At times like this, some people even stop believing in the "calories in vs. calories out" concept. It doesn't seem true anymore, but it is. Don't ever, ever question "calories in vs. calories out." It should be the one truth that you can cling to in your weight-loss quest. If you lose sight of that, you're sunk!

Interestingly enough, the concept of "calories in vs. calories out" is usually the culprit of the weight loss plateau. Before you get really angry, try to remember that a concept based on math and biology really isn't capable of spontaneously making exceptions just so that your life is easier.

But how can "calories in vs. calories out" be the cause, when you used to lose weight by eating the same things and doing the same exercise that you do now? Let's break this down. Suppose you are a 250-pound man who has already lost thirty pounds at a good healthy rate of one pound per week. You have been walking for forty minutes a day, have been getting in 10,000 steps daily, and have been eating more fruits and vegetables. You continue to do all of these things exactly as you have since you started this process about thirty weeks ago, but the results have come to a halt. You are now in the dreaded plateau stage.

Think of all of the ways that your body burns calories. The main ones are basal metabolism and physical activity. When you man started out, you weighed 250 pounds. You are now at 220 pounds. A 250-pound body has a higher basal metabolism than a 220-pound body. There is just more body to maintain when you weigh thirty pounds more. A forty minute long walk is more difficult for a 250-pound body than a 220-pound body, so the 250-pound body burns more calories during a walk of the exact same length. As a 250-pound body takes steps throughout the day, each step requires more effort than a step taken by a 220-pound body. So in your new 220-pound body, you are doing less exercise with each movement in the day, and you also need fewer calories each day to maintain yourself. Because of this, you are no longer putting yourself into a calorie deficit each day. The changes in calories burned during the walk and in calories burned through basal metabolism and daily movement have entirely eaten up your calorie debt. Your daily calorie equation has now become balanced. It doesn't seem fair, but it is true. This might be disheartening, but try to be optimistic. You are only in this predicament because you successfully lost weight in the first place. Good job.

You originally lost weight due to your ability to use up more calories than you were consuming. The fantastic news is that this logic still completely applies to your situation. Your calorie-burning capacity during any given activity has diminished somewhat, but this isn't a bad thing. Your heart and other organs are not working as hard when you go about your daily activities or when you walk up a flight of stairs. Life is probably a little more comfortable in your new body, and that's great! Congratulations.

Now to continue on the path to weight loss, you have to repeat the steps that you did the first time you started the whole weight loss business. If you are currently maintaining, then you can assume that your calorie equation is balanced. Re-evaluate your activity and nutrition. You will have to continue what you are already doing, plus bump it up a notch or two. You could add another ten minutes on to your daily walk. You could just pick up the pace while you walk for the forty minutes. You could add in some more steps. The options are endless, just like the first time. Pick something that won't be too hard for you to maintain, just like the first changes that you made.

Because this process is familiar to you, it should be easier this time. You may have already discovered some things that do and do not work for you when trying to adjust your calorie equation. If something worked the first time, do it again. Tweak your habits the same way you did when you started this process. Increase physical activity whenever you can. Cut out a few calories where you won't miss them. There is no need for originality here. Stick with things that work and that you enjoy.

If you again implement those little changes that affect your overall calorie balance for the day, you will again begin to see weight loss. You may hit another plateau in another twenty or thirty or forty pounds, but you will know what to do.

Keep in mind that it is perfectly acceptable to take a "break" from weight loss and maintain your weight at a set point for a while. Creating that daily calorie deficit requires work, more work than maintaining a calorie balance, and sometimes in life you don't have that extra energy. If you come up against some really big personal obstacles in your life that take a lot of your energy, allow yourself to maintain your weight until you have the time to invest in continuing the weight loss process.

Another important thing to do is to remind yourself why you care. Why are you trying to lose weight? What is the point of all of this trouble that you are going to? After working at something for a long time, it becomes harder to see the big picture and easier to get mired down in the day-to-day trouble that you are causing yourself. It's easy to lose that initial enthusiasm after you have been blasting away at your goal for awhile. You probably have a lot of good reasons for wanting to lose weight, so don't let those slip out of your mind!

Different people find different methods helpful for remembering their goals. For some, written reminders tucked in personal places are the best. You might find a little note to yourself in your desk or in your bedroom dresser drawer. The messages don't even have to be written words. Pictures, sketches, or any sort of code that you may have worked out with yourself will do just fine. The important thing is that you have a reminder of the reason behind your weight loss goals.

Alternately, Some people don't do very well with subtle reminders. They don't easily absorb this kind of communication. These are the people who will tape bright or sarcastic messages their doors so that they cannot ignore themselves. If this style is the best for you, you will probably know recognize it without too much thought.

Engaging other people close to you in your weight loss goals can be helpful as well. You can brief a friend on the reasons you want to lose weight and tell him or her to remember those reasons for when you ask later. If you should happen to call this person later on when you are feeling frustrated and grouchy about the whole topic, he or she will remind you why you are putting yourself through this. Of course, this technique only works for those who have a trustworthy friend who lets them call and complain about things like this.

If you are the kind of person that finds certain books, movies, songs, or articles inspiring, you could keep some of those things around to pump you up when you need it most. If Rocky is the only one who gets you feeling good enough to go do your exercise, then pull it out as necessary. You don't have to actually admit to anyone that that's why you own the boxed set. It's for your own benefit.

At the very, very least, mentally identify your personal reasons for losing weight. Maybe you want your knees to feel better. You are sick of them getting sore every day after just a little walking. Maybe you just want to save some money on your health and life insurance premiums. Maybe your goal is to be around and healthy for your kids' kids. These are worthy goals. You will find your own personal reasons more inspiring than anyone else's reasons, so think up some of your own. Write them down. Think of them when weight loss gets hard.

As obstacles come up, address the source of each one. Take it day by day. Ask yourself, " Can I move my calorie equation in my favor for today?" Do that today and then ask yourself about it again tomorrow. You are in this for the long haul, so challenges will come up, but you can overcome them all (even if you have to wear out the Rocky tapes in the process.)

CHAPTER 12

How to Maintain your Ideal Weight

If you have gone through the long and arduous weight loss process and have arrived at your ideal weight, congratulations! You have assessed your eating habits and activity habits. You have cut calories here and there. You have increased your steps and your daily minutes of physical activity. Through all of these changes, you have managed to achieve the goal that you started out with, which was to lose a certain amount of pounds to improve your health.

The hardest part is done. Now all you have to do to maintain the weight that you have reached is to balance your daily calorie intake with your daily calorie output. Months and months of having to create a daily calorie deficit have made you very good at manipulating your calories. Balancing is even easier than making the calorie deficit.

Even though maintaining weight loss is easier than losing weight, it is a good thing to remember that it does still require some level of effort on your part. If you stop paying any sort of attention to maintaining your weight loss, or if you drift back into your old habits, it is extremely likely that you will gain back some, if not all, of the weight that you have worked so hard to lose. Many people even gain extra weight back after they have lost a few pounds.

The good news is that this does not have to be the case with you. You have lost your weight in a very healthy fashion, which puts you at an advantage to begin with. The healthy weight loss process has also taught you a thing or two that you can remember for the future. You have the tools to survive this test. Maintenance involves the application and the reapplication of all of the tricks you know to stay active, eat well, and balance that calorie equation.

Weight maintenance demands that you continue doing all of the things that you have done for weight loss. Except that now you will do them permanently. "Permanently" as in the rest of your life. That doesn't have to sound so ominous. It's good to identify your intent from the start. You want to maintain this weight loss forever, correct?

The time frame you are working with makes it all the more vital that you have made changes that you can live with. Hopefully you have made changes that you enjoy, and that make you feel good. If this is not the case, now is a very good time to reevaluate your choices. Say you have lost twenty pounds by using a stepper in your basement every night. You kind of hate doing it, but it was motivating because you could see the results as the weight came off.

If you are in this situation and you stop doing the stepper, you could gain weight back because that is a fair amount of calories that you were burning each day. On the other hand, you really dislike the stepper and probably aren't going to be able to do it for the rest of your life. This situation is definitely headed in a bad direction. Don't start out your weight maintenance plan like this!

Make adjustments where necessary. You are certainly allowed to switch working out on the stepper for any other type of calorie-burning activity that you do so desire. The options are endless. Extensive discussion of physical activity and exercise options occurred in previous chapters. You know what you like; switch to it. You could also make another adjustment to your eating habits to compensate for the reduction in exercise. Exercise has health benefits that go beyond weight loss, however, so try to continue doing something. Also, most people find that exercise and/or physical activity makes weight maintenance much, much easier.

If you feel that everything is in good order now, great. Continue with the status quo until you run into problems. Maybe you used to walk with some coworkers every day at lunch. This was your tried-and-true weight maintenance plan, and you enjoyed it.

A couple of years later, you switched jobs. Your new coworkers don't believe in exercise, and the office is not at all situated so that you can take walks anyway. At this point you would need to make another adjustment. Remember that you are still in weight maintenance! Some changes will be out of your control, but you still need to adjust for them when they come up.

Weight maintenance is essentially eternally making small adjustments. Life is very dynamic. What works well at this point in your life might not be the best thing next month or ten years from now. Be flexible. The important thing is to maintain your weight loss, not to maintain a rigid routine that never changes.

Another important concept is to maintain overall balance. Ideally, you would be able to maintain a perfect balance for every single day for the rest of your life. If you have been alive for any length of time already, you may have noticed that life isn't really like that. There are all kinds of changes and ups and downs. Christmas comes and you eat more cookies. Summer comes and you get more outdoor activity. Different phases in your life are different.

Individual situations also have a way of wreaking havoc on your body weight. Maybe you go on a 10-day cruise for your anniversary. On any good cruise you end up eating restaurant food about five times a day. This is probably not going to come as a surprise for you. From the minute that you started saving money for the vacation, you figured that it would probably turn out this way. In a case like this, try to maintain the best balance possible while on vacation, but plan ahead of time for this minor bump in your weight maintenance path.

You could be sure to be very active the week before your vacation. Take every opportunity to maintain high activity levels while on vacation as well. Vacations are usually a great opportunity for new and exciting kinds of exercise and physical activity in a completely fresh environment. After you get back home, know that you will probably be eating even a little lighter and exercising a little more than usual until you have fully recovered from your vacation eating habits.

There are an endless amount of situations that could affect you in a similar way. Say you are going right along with your daily exercise program and lifting weights. You are feeling pretty buff in general and on top of the world. February comes and you end up catching the flu. It's a bad year for it, so you have to stay home from work for a week because you are so miserable. Even after you start working again, it is a couple more weeks until you feel like yourself again. Through this whole month, you haven't done any of your exercises at all. Once you return to your weights, you find that you can't lift as much as before. You also can't do any cardiovascular exercise at the same speed that you were used to. You just feel a little more wiped out than before.

This situation is common and will probably happen to you more than once if you plan to maintain your activity for the rest of your life. A couple of weeks of illness seems to really undo some of the things you have been working on. It is at this point that you need to remember that you are maintaining. Don't beat yourself up for a week or two off of your exercise schedule, whether it was due to illness or an extra project at work. Just get back on track as quickly as possible after you are derailed. Work yourself back up to where you were before. Be concerned about the big picture, not the one week that you missed for a very good reason.

In this way, you maintain balance over time even though you have not balanced out each individual day. Realistically, you won't be able to avoid every single instance of under-exercising or overeating for the rest of your life, so you'd better just be as reasonable as possible and be ready to compensate when it does happen. It's the only way that your weight loss is going to be able to survive the ups and downs of life.

Over the decades you will also experience biological changes that will require adjustments in your eating and exercising. Every ten years after age thirty you will be losing a couple hundred calories or so per day because your basal metabolism slows down. This is not a huge change, and if you are truly maintaining, it will be easy to roll with the punches. Expect some things to change somewhere in the future and know that you are going to do what it takes to survive the changes.

Small adjustments over time are the essence of maintenance.

Think of the word "maintenance" in the general sense. If you are maintaining something, that implies that it is already in good shape. It doesn't need repairs; this is no fixer-upper. The only objective of maintenance is to preserve the current good state of whatever it is that you are maintaining.

Think about what maintenance typically requires. There are going to be a few minor replacements, some cleaning tasks, and a lot of preventative measures taken. You do the little things as you go along to prevent bigger problems. Think of some things that you personally maintain. Maybe you maintain a house or a vehicle of some kind.

In the case of a house, maintenance includes painting and repainting, cleaning windows, and getting the leaves out of the gutters. You might need to do various tests in your house to make sure there are no problems. You pay people to check for termites or to check on the furnace. You realize that paying a little bit to avoid problems is a lot less hassle and cost than having to get a whole new house. It makes sense. If you abandon your house until it is in such bad shape that it is condemned, it is going to be a whole lot more work to get it looking good.

In the case of a car or truck, maintenance includes regular oil and filter changes, replacing spark plugs every so often, tune-ups, and tire rotations. You replace various fluids as you run out of them and little lights go on all over the dashboard. If you hear a weird sound one day, you pop the hood right away to see what could be wrong. You do this to keep the engine running well. You want to avoid having to buy another car anytime soon. You also don't want to run the risk of getting stranded one day on the side of the road because something important suddenly failed due to your lack of care.

Maintenance requirements for your body and your weight loss are not really so different from the requirements for buildings and vehicles. The main difference between the two is that cars and houses can be replaced, but if you mess up big time with your body, there is not nearly as much that you can do to correct the situation. You can't tear down and rebuild, as much as it sometimes seems like a good idea.

There are some regular, daily things you need to do to maintain your body. Daily actions required are eating and moving. Balancing your calorie equation is a daily task as well. There are other, Less frequently needed actions too. Every week or so you may check in on your weight to make sure that it is the same. If you need adjustments, they can be made at this time to correct for any problems. You visit your primary care physician for annual physicals to make sure that all is well. Corrections could be made at this point too, as needed. Clearing up a small infection or a tendency towards high blood pressure when it first begins results in avoidance of potential major health issues.

The entire concept of maintenance is to take care of the little things before compounding little things morph into one big thing. In this way you make life a lot easier for yourself. You don't come equipped with warning lights, but think of some of the signs that you see when you are physically headed in the wrong direction.

You may feel a little more sluggish than usual. Maybe certain articles of clothing begin to fit you a little tighter. If your weight changes on the scale, or your body fat percentage increases, or you have to use the next hole on your belt, these all serve as warning signs that some maintenance is needed immediately to avoid bigger problems.

Try to remember to utilize whatever method you prefer for measuring your weight. Be sure to continue to assess your body weight even after you have lost all that you want to lose. Now is the time to make sure that you have kept off what you have already lost.

If you previously weighed yourself each week, or each month as you lost weight, don't abandon that practice during the weight maintenance stage. Daily weighing isn't recommended during weight loss because you don't see much change, but some people like to weigh themselves every day after they have reached their ideal weight. It becomes part of their daily routine. They may brush their teeth, then weigh themselves, then get in the shower, then get dressed for work, etc. It's just part of the day. In this way, it is easier to see the earliest warning sign when it comes up.

You may have maintained your weight successfully for ten years, when one day you notice that you have gained a pound or two. This is your cue to kick into maintenance mode. For the next couple of days, try to get your calorie equation to come out with a net loss. Increase your activity and decrease your calories consumed. In a week or so you will have completely taken care of the problem and be back to normal That is your damage control system at its finest. This maintenance process can be repeated over and over again as needed.

Figure out what "alarms" are most noticeable and helpful for you. Most likely there are several things that will change in your body when you gain a couple of pounds. If you are tuned in to what is happening, you will see the alarms. When those alarms ring, take immediate action to correct the problem . Adjust the little things as you go along to maintain your weight permanently. You can successfully maintain your weight. You thoroughly understand "calories in vs. calories out." You have learned to work the concept to your advantage to get the results that you want. Don't give up now. You have worked so hard to get to your ideal weight; don't let it slip back away from you!

2078282R00068

Printed in Great Britain
by Amazon.co.uk, Ltd.,
Marston Gate.